FIXING THE PRIMARY CARE CRISIS

ADVANCE PRAISE FOR FIXING THE PRIMARY CARE CRISIS

"Steve Schimpff has written an outstanding treatise describing how misdirected attempts to save money have underfunded primary care resulting in lower quality healthcare, an increasing shortage of primary care physicians, and an increase in the cost of healthcare. He shows how a change in the healthcare paradigm can lead to better care at lower cost that is more rewarding to patient and physician."

—*Robert J. Alpern, MD Ensign Professor of Medicine and Dean, Yale School of Medicine*

"With nearly 3000 employees, the health of our company depends on a healthy workforce. We deliver highly-advanced technical and engineering services, so illnesses, as well as the cost and quality of healthcare available to our employees, directly impact our productivity and customer satisfaction. *Fixing the Primary Care Crisis* brings attention to an issue that will resonate with businesses of every size, in any market."

—*Bahman Atefi, ScD, CEO, Alion Science and Technology*

"Dr. Schimpff eloquently illustrates one of the principle lessons we teach our medical students throughout their training: relationship matters. He rightly asks how the doctor-patient relationship has suffered in today's medical/commerce environment. Dr. Schimpff's powerful patient vignettes and wide ranging interviews provide thought provoking concerns for physicians, patients and those of us whose mission is to train the next generation of healthcare providers."

—*Robert A. Barish, MD MBA, Chancellor, LSU Health Sciences Center, Shreveport*

"*Fixing The Primary Care Crisis* is an outstanding work by an extraordinary writer. As in his previous works, Dr. Schimpff has clearly identified the issue in a manner for all to understand. The crisis is real and imminent and we would all be served in heeding Steve's advice."

—*Stephen Burch, Chairman of the Board, University of Maryland Medical System, former president, Atlantic Division, Comcast Inc. and retired CEO, Virgin Media UK*

FIXING THE PRIMARY CARE CRISIS

RECLAIMING THE PATIENT-DOCTOR RELATIONSHIP AND RETURNING HEALTHCARE DECISIONS TO YOU AND YOUR DOCTOR

Stephen C. Schimpff, MD FACP

For
Carol
My best friend, lover and soul mate

Our daughter and son-in-law
Becky and Brian
Who make us proud

Our grandsons
Ben and Bruno
Who bring us joy

TABLE OF CONTENTS

FOREWORD

A Nation in Search of Healthcare Solutions

How did it come to this? How is it possible for a nation that is the world's wealthiest and most powerful, with reams of data on hand and with an abundance of MBAs to analyze them, to produce arguably the advanced world's most inefficient healthcare system?

The statistics are sobering. America spends about 18 percent of its GDP on healthcare, yet we hardly look like a nation that devotes nearly a fifth of its resources to physical and mental well-being. As a telling example, only a handful of nations are as diabetic as we are, and most of them are tiny ones like Netherlands Antilles, Tonga, and Nauru. According to the CDC, nearly 10 percent of Americans are diabetic.

Not coincidentally, more than a third of us are obese, which contributes both to the prevalence of diabetes and to healthcare spending. By 2008, the estimated annual medical cost of obesity in the U.S. was approaching $150 billion, roughly twice the level of cost one decade earlier. Almost half of that cost was borne by Medicare and Medicaid.

Our hearts are literally breaking. Approximately 600,000 people die of heart disease every year – about 1 in 4 deaths. Each year, about 720,000 of us have a heart attack (a disproportionate share are probably Bears fans). Coronary heart disease costs the U.S. about $110 billion per year according to the CDC. The best that can be said about the situation is that heart disease fails to discriminate. It is the leading cause of death for most ethnicities in the U.S. including African-Americans, whites, and Hispanics.

If anything, we should be the envy of the world. After all, we create most of the world's breakthrough medical technologies. According to the Pharmaceutical Research and Manufacturers Association, American companies conduct the majority of the world's research and development in pharmaceuticals and hold the intellectual property rights on most new medicines. According to the Commerce Department, the biopharmaceutical pipeline is in the midst of developing more than 5,000 new medicines with approximately 3,400 compounds being studied in America, more than any other region in the world.

So with all that expenditure and innovation, we should live happily ever after, or at least happily for a long time. But we are not that happy. According to a recent ranking of world happiness, we Americans are neither as happy as our neighbors to the north in Canada or to the south in Mexico. What's more, those countries aren't nearly as happy as the world's center of joy, Scandinavia.

The good news is that because we die earlier than others, our misery does not last as long as it otherwise would. According to the World Health Organization (2012), Japan boasts the world's longest life expectancy at about 85 years. Other nations that rank high on the list include Singapore, Iceland, Italy, Sweden, Australia, Canada, Switzerland, Spain, Israel, France, Norway, Austria, the Netherlands, Ireland, and the U.K. At under 80 years, we rank below Lebanon and Slovenia.

Here's what's truly amazing – our circumstances are about to deteriorate. How can this be you ask given the Affordable Care Act and the broadening of insurance coverage across the land? Simple – the marketplace isn't positioned to support sustained improvement in outcomes and the public sector lacks the resources necessary to chip in enough resources.

A recent Medicare Trustees' report indicates that the insolvency date for the Hospital Insurance trust fund is 2026. For its part, Medicaid has wreaked havoc on both federal and state budgets for years. According to data released by the Department of Health and Human Services, one in five Americans now receive their health insurance through a state Medicaid program.

To improve outcomes, some American policymakers have adopted the position that more timely intervention will both improve healthcare outcomes and save money. Makes sense, until one thinks through the economics. At the heart of the new American health paradigm is the primary care physician – the medical point guard who takes control early in the shot clock and distributes the ball to specialists on an as-needed basis.

But there's a big difference between the NBA point guard and the primary care physician. NBA point guards are paid handsomely. Take Chris Paul of the LA Clippers. He earns more than $21 million a year, while Derrick Rose of the Chicago Bulls earns nearly $19 million and John Wall of the Washington Wizards takes home pre-tax earnings approaching $17 million. Among the 14 highest paid players in the NBA, four are point guards. Only small forwards are as well represented among the best paid players.

The primary care physician, by contrast, is a pauper in relative terms. Colleagues that go on to specialize as cardiothoracic surgeons or dermatologists receive median salaries of $525,944 and $411,499, respectively. The median salary for primary care physicians is roughly $220,000.

Money isn't everything of course, but one needs to at least pay back their debts. According to the Association of American Medical Colleges, the median cost of medical school attendance for the Class of 2015 exceeds $226,000 for public universities (in-state) and nearly $300,000 for those attending private universities.

No wonder that in order to meet the demand for medical services last year, the U.S. would have required 9,000 more primary care physicians. The implementation of the Affordable Care Act and the ongoing aging of America will only make the situation worse.

One might be tempted to suggest that more money could solve this issue, but from where would that funding emerge over the many years to come? As of this writing, America has already amassed a nation debt exceeding $18 trillion and will have a difficult time simply funding current Medicare, Social Security, education, defense, and homeland security service levels.

Even if there were enough physicians, would they really be able to diagnose diseases and manage treatment during the 8-12 minutes they spend with each patient? If anything, as physician shortages worsen, the time physicians spend with their patients will decline even further.

These short visits result from a financially lethal combination of inadequate reimbursement and rising overhead and liability costs. The primary care physician has little choice but to shore up her/his business model by striving for volume. Incredibly, the lack of "face time" with patients results in greater healthcare utilization, not less. Not only are diagnoses more likely to be missed leading to higher numbers of ER visits, but the primary care physician, wracked with uncertainty, ends up ordering more tests and referring patients to specialists "just in case." All of this drives up the health system's costs, wastes time for both patient are caregiver, and produces suboptimal healthcare outcomes.

Some of these primary care physicians are likely to move toward a concierge model in which they see a smaller pool of patients who are willing to pay a premium for their service. Some might call them greedy, but this also represents a realistic manner by which these physicians will be able to provide patient-centered care that looks more like traditional medicine and less like the service sector's version of a fast-paced assembly line.

A Better, Simpler, More Elegant Approach to the Delivery of Primary Care

The situation appears hopeless, but it is not. There are solutions and Dr. Stephen C Schimpff offers them up neatly in *Fixing The Primary Care Crisis*.

The fact of the matter is that the primary care physician (PCP) needs more time with each patient, not less. How can this be achieved under the current regime? The answer is that it cannot be.

That's what makes Dr. Schimpff's book such a revelation. There are innovative approaches that can be supported by PCPs, insurers, employers, and the public sector and Dr. Schimpff walks us through many of them. Oddly enough, at the heart of these new approaches aren't people in lab coats and ties, but patients themselves.

Patients will need to advocate for one another, to call out for refinements in the delivery and financing of care, and influence legislators and implementers alike. It will take a grassroots effort to transform America's healthcare system and Dr. Schimpff explains the role that each of us will need to play if we are to live healthier, longer, and within our means.

At the heart of the healthcare system's problems is that it is far too complex. There are too many bureaucrats, regulators, insurance brokers, hospital administrators, codes, tests, machine manufacturers, salespeople, and politicians abroad. The key is to take a deep breath and simplify.

This is precisely the approach that Dr. Schimpff adopts. As an internist/researcher/professor/healthcare CEO and all-around Renaissance man, Dr. Schimpff lays out an elegant plan that both administrator and care deliverer can follow. His is a new paradigm – one that values the experiences of both patient and provider while rationalizing the use of scarce resources.

Anirban Basu
CEO and economist, Sage Policy Group, Inc.
Baltimore, MD

Anirban Basu is an economist, lawyer, professor, business owner, journalist, consultant and public speaker. He holds graduate degrees in economics, law and public policy. In 2004, he founded Sage Policy Group, Inc., a consultancy located in downtown Baltimore with clients in more than 40 states and in several countries. He is also a principal at Sage Growth Partners, a healthcare consultancy located on the other side of Baltimore's Inner Harbor. He currently lectures at the Johns Hopkins University in Global Strategy where he has also taught micro-, macro-, international and urban economics.

PREFACE: A RETURN TO RELATIONSHIP MEDICINE

Susan* is 56, married, insured, a successful professional and is in generally good health. She began to have a strange sensation in her right chest, which she described as a shooting sensation almost electrical or vibrational in nature which stretches from high up in her right chest down as a narrow line over her rib cage and onto her abdomen. It seems to be immediately under the skin, starts intermittently and ends at no set time. She visited her primary care physician (PCP) and gave this description, adding that she was concerned that it might be her heart. The doctor asked additional questions and did an exam and electrocardiogram. All were normal except for the description of the sensation Susan was feeling.

Her PCP was now running out of time for the fifteen minute visit. Here was a fork in the road with two paths. Given that Susan indicated a concern about her heart, the PCP chose the path to send her to a cardiologist for further evaluation. The cardiologist did a history and exam related to her heart and found nothing abnormal but suggested a stress test and an echocardiogram. Both were normal. The cardiologist said it was not Susan's heart causing the problem, but since the sensation crossed over to the upper abdomen, maybe it would be a good idea to see a gastroenterologist. The GI doctor also did a history and exam and found nothing. Nevertheless, among many other tests, he ordered a CT scan of the abdomen. All was normal except for a small cyst in her uterus. The radiologist

---

* Here and with other patient stories in this book, the individual's name and other identifying information have been changed to assure anonymity and given just as a first name. Doctors' names that are given as a first and last name are real; those given just as last names only refer to doctors who wished their comments to be anonymous.

read it as a benign cyst but – feeling the need to be cautious – recommended Susan visit a gynecologist. The gynecologist also said it looked benign, but to be on the safe side, she could remove it laproscopically. Susan would be "out of the hospital the same day and feeling fine in a day or so." The cyst was just that, a benign cyst.

Susan still had the strange sensation in her chest and no one had found an answer for her. But given that it seemed to have an electrical feeling, the gynecologist suggested that it could be a nerve issue. So she visited a neurologist who found nothing, commenting that nerves run around the chest, not up and down.

Susan's story illustrates the problem so common today in primary care. The primary care physician should be the backbone of the American healthcare system. But primary care is in crisis – a very serious crisis. In this story, the PCP did not truly listen to his patient. He did not stop and think the issue out carefully. He had no time to delve into what might actually cause Susan's pain since there was a waiting room full of patients and he needed to see about 25 that day. So instead, he took the easier path and referred the patient to a cardiologist since this seemed like a logical choice. Had he followed the other side of the fork in the road, listened long enough and then thought about it, he would have concluded that Susan was hypersensitive to minor – albeit real – sensations. He would have offered reassurance that it did not represent a life-threatening ailment. He would have said that it was real but of no concern. He might have offered a few weeks of a low-dose anti-anxiety medication such as alprazolam (Xanax), offered further reassurance and told her to return in two weeks for a follow-up. At the follow-up, he might have explored the issues producing anxiety or stress in her life – finances, marital relationship, a disruptive child, or an overbearing in-law.[†] What Susan really needed was assistance to overcome her stress, not months

---

† After hearing about this patient's saga, I asked a highly-regarded PCP to comment on how he would have cared for this patient. I told him only about the initial visit. He smiled and said, "I bet she got sent for a big workup." He then offered his approach, which I have reiterated in the story. But not everyone would agree. A gerontologist, after reading the entire story, suggested that Xanax is highly addictive and he would have avoided it, especially in an older person, instead relying on personal   interaction alone with the patient. A cardiologist pointed out that women often present with atypical cardiac pain. He would have done the echocardiogram and the stress test just to be sure there was no heart problem.

of specialist hopping, which was unnecessary, expensive and only increased her stress.

Anxiety and stress are often components associated with a physical symptom, and these can only be addressed with more time to carefully listen and respond with suggestions. But Susan was shipped from doctor to doctor, test to test, and even had an operation with no one really listening enough to figure out her problem. All each specialist could do was say it was not in his or her "organ system" and leave her without a sense of closure. Each said it was not the heart, the stomach or the nerves. And the surgery "went fine," but she still had the unpleasant sensation. All of this resulted in far less than adequate medical care and cost a king's ransom. That is what happens today. All that was needed was for the PCP to spend some more time – time to listen, then to think and then to counsel. That's not expensive at all.

Susan's story and her travails with the medical system illustrate how deep the problem goes. Her journey highlights the issues that drove me to research and write this book. Multiple other patient vignettes scattered throughout the book will underscore the reality of the crisis – and its impact on all of us. In the process, I will explain how you, as a patient, can receive excellent care at limited expense.

The Argument Defined

Why do primary care physicians have so little time? The short answer is our insurance system, which attempts to manage costs through price controls. For years, Medicare has set a low reimbursement rate for regular office visits to a patient's PCP. Commercial insurance always follows Medicare's lead and has done likewise. As a result, reimbursement rates have remained fairly steady for a decade, even as office costs have risen each year. With costs rising and income steady, PCPs are forced to make up the difference through volume. This means seeing more patients per day, usually about 25 (and often more). In order to see that many, the PCP generally stops seeing his or her patients in the hospital or ER and shortens the time per visit to about 10-12 minutes of actual "face time" with the patient. In inflation adjusted dollars, a PCP earns somewhat less today than in 1970 yet sees about twice as many patients per day. PCPs have been forced to focus on quantity when they should focus on quality.

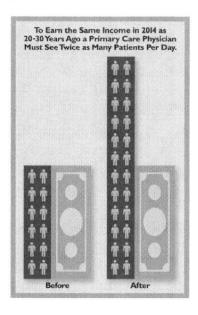

This has created a serious dilemma in primary care. Individual primary care physicians have a panel of patients (the number of patients they serve) that is too large for quality comprehensive primary care. At the same time, the U.S. is experiencing a primary care physician shortage. This combination of too few PCPs serving too many patients means that primary care is not what it should be.

When they do have time, PCPs can treat the vast majority of issues brought to them by their patients without the need for specialist referrals or excessive testing. They can – and do – give superb preventive care. This care reduces serious chronic illnesses in the future, especially for the diseases that today account for 75-85 percent of all medical costs. When PCPs do have time, they can handle 90 percent (or more) of the care needs of those with chronic illnesses without a specialist referral. They can coordinate the care of patients who do need to be referred, ensuring high levels of quality at a reasonable cost. By doing this, they can develop a trusting relationship and be true healers.

To be clear, I do not fault the PCPs. They have been pushed into this model of care, kicking and screaming and with the sense that there is no escape. Their frustrations are high, primarily because they know and feel that they could serve you better if they only had more time to do so.

This crisis is the most pressing and urgent issue in healthcare delivery today. Healthcare delivery must be restructured now so that everyone, especially older adults with multiple chronic illnesses, can obtain quality, compassionate and cost effective care. This means having a committed primary care doctor who has the *time,* along with the knowledge and experience, to deliver the care needed. This will require both a change in how primary care is delivered *and* how it is purchased.

Time, or the lack of it, is the single biggest issue facing PCPs in our healthcare system. It means quality of care is less than it should be, costs are too high and the opportunity for true healing is remote. It is impossible to deliver high quality care in a 10-15 minute visit when the patient has three to five chronic illnesses, is taking multiple prescription medications, and presents his PCP with a new symptom. Likewise, it is impossible without adequate time to deliver humane care to patients who have stress and anxiety as underlying or contributing factors to an illness. If a patient arrives with a symptom slightly out of the ordinary, as Susan did, the primary care physician currently has no time to figure out the underlying issue. The PCP punts by referring patients to a specialist and ordering numerous tests and X-rays. This, of course, greatly increases total costs, often without positively impacting the patient.

The result is that patients feel the primary care physician is not listening to them, that there are far too many tests and specialty referrals that do little to improve care, and that the costs are high. This is all definitely true. Everyone is frustrated and no one – patient, doctor or insurer – is satisfied. Each is frustrated for different reasons: The patient is not getting answers, the doctor is overworked, and the insurance company is not profitable enough.

This outcome is the inevitable result of making primary care an unattractive, second-rate career option in medicine today and producing the PCP shortage. It is a conundrum with a vicious downward spiral leading to a serious crisis. Primary care physicians are leaving private practices in droves to work for the local hospital or retiring early, if possible. Medical students see that primary care physicians are running on a treadmill yet earn half as much as most specialists despite their heavy responsibilities and busy schedules, so they choose other medical career paths. There is now a shortage of primary care physicians, and it will only be exacerbated in the coming years. Today America has about 30 percent PCPs, down substantially from decades ago and far below the PCP-to-specialist ratio of 70 percent/30 percent in almost every other developed country.

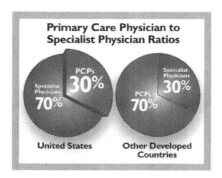

Plus, today about 9 percent of all visits to PCPs result in a specialist referral, far higher than necessary. This is up from about 5 percent a decade earlier, with 41 million referrals then compared to 105 million in 2010. The growth was faster for PCPs working in a large hospital or hospital system. Medicare enrollee referral rates more than doubled and, combined with more total Medicare enrollee PCP visits, the total increase in referrals was greater than 350 percent.[1]

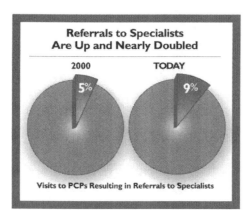

You – as a patient caught in this crisis who is seeking quality healthcare – will need to educate yourself about what you can do to ensure you receive outstanding primary care. Throughout this book, you will learn that there are other options to secure quality healthcare, all which require you to assume a more direct relationship with your PCP. We will explore options that include direct primary care-based practices, which feature a much better PCP-to-patient ratio. In these practices, a PCP has a more realistic patient load between 500 and 800 patients (versus the more typical 2,500 or more). This enables the physician to offer same or next-day appointments for as long as necessary (versus today's 15 minutes), 24/7 access via cell phone and a return to real "relationship-based medicine."

These practices, often referred to as retainer-based, concierge or membership, have been criticized as only for the "1 percent," but this is a misnomer. A monthly fee of about $75 ($900 per year) is common, with some charging substantially less. Since you are paying the doctor directly, the "business relationship" changes and the PCP is highly motivated to seek ways to keep your expenses as low as possible and consistent with the best possible healthcare. Many direct primary care doctors make generic medications available at wholesale prices, which further reduces costs and may offset the entire cost of the membership for those taking many medications. Many doctors also offer access to highly-discounted laboratory testing with the premier national laboratories and reduced imaging at local radiology practices. The result is more money in your pocket *and* much better healthcare.

Some employers are recognizing that they can offer a high-deductible policy and concurrently pay the retainer for the direct primary care physician. Thus, they get comprehensive primary care services for their employees because they understand the *economic* benefits of the right doctor-to-patient ratio and how more time with patients can actually improve their employees' health, which leads to greater productivity and reduced insurance premiums in the coming years. A win-win for employer and employee and a return to real "relationship-based medicine."

The dollars spent on *primary care* will be more than the current 5 percent of total health care costs, perhaps about 7-9 percent. But the result will be better care – by far – with greater satisfaction for patient and doctor alike. Most importantly, there will be a major reduction in the *total costs of care*, leading to satisfaction for insurers, employers and you as well. Not only will you be healthier, but you will save money with fewer visits to specialists, fewer tests and fewer prescriptions. The resolution is not one of adding money to the system but of reallocating the money, which will ultimately reduce total expenditures.

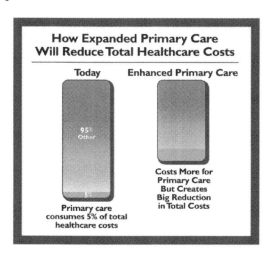

How Expanded Primary Care Will Reduce Total Healthcare Costs

Today — 95% Other / 5% — Primary care consumes 5% of total healthcare costs

Enhanced Primary Care — Costs More for Primary Care But Creates Big Reduction in Total Costs

What is needed is innovation. That never comes from above. It comes from the front lines. It will come from you and your physician. It will come from enlightened employers who see healthcare as a strategic priority rather than only a cost. It will come from insurers that realize the old ways do not work. It will come from newly-forming organizations that perceive a new pathway. It will come from retail stores that see a potential advantage for their businesses. Some innovations will be successful, and some will not. But the best will survive, and with them, a new era will develop. An era with better health and lower costs.

Although it makes little sense to pine for the days gone by, it is true that most of the "old time" general practitioners were healers. My grandfather graduated from medical school in the late 1890s and set up practice in an office attached to his home. Patients lined up on the wrap around porch and waited their turn. He took whatever time seemed appropriate. He had few drugs, few tests to run and a limited surgical armamentarium. But his patients knew that he cared, that he listened to them, and that he understood their cares and sorrows. When he went to a home to deliver a baby, his payment was often pulled from under the mattress, saved up during the pregnancy. Often patients could not pay, and instead they brought him a bushel of potatoes when their harvest came in. It was a simpler time without the wealth of advantages we have today, yet he was revered as the town healer. We cannot and should not go back to the past, but there are aspects of those times that do need to be continued and nurtured today.

Book and Author Background

To develop this book, I conducted in-depth interviews that lasted about an hour and covered 22 specific questions with many primary care physicians. Most are in private practice and a few are in an academic setting; some are internists and others family physicians; some are men and some women; some have been in practice for a long time and some are only recently beginning their careers. There are a number of patient stories included. The stories are real, with names and other identifying data changed to protect their anonymity. In addition, I interviewed multiple other doctors with questions directed at one or more specific issues raised by the initial interviews. I have also tapped my contacts built up over a long career to ascertain various perspectives from around the country and from multiple venues. I have looked back on the more than 150 interviews done for *The Future of Health Care Delivery,* and I have used my own 50 years of clinical, management and leadership experience and observations of healthcare delivery, including my time as COO of a hospital system and then CEO of an academic medical center.

A word about myself: I am not a primary care physician. I was trained and am board certified in internal medicine, medical oncology and infectious diseases. My clinical career was with patients who had leukemia or lymphoma and with the serious infections that befall those receiving aggressive cancer chemotherapy. I did, however, often serve as the de facto primary care physician for many of my long-time patients. This combination of personal experiences over a long career, coupled with intensive direct research over the past few years, has led to this book. Because I am not a primary care physician, I am able to provide a balanced look at the issues discussed – and provide solutions that work for everyone involved: patient, physician, insurer, and employer.

Let me be clear. I do have an agenda. It is to transform primary care in a manner that allows the primary care physician to offer his or her patients the best care in a cost effective manner that improves quality yet reduces the total costs of care. This transformation is long overdue. This book will educate, motivate and call to action everyone involved for the transformation to take place.

With this terribly dysfunctional healthcare system that exists today, it is imperative that you understand what outstanding primary care is, what it can mean for your health and what adverse settings the typical PCP endures today. It is imperative that you become an active proponent for change. Physicians cannot do it alone, and it is evident that government will not be the change agent. Effective and lasting improvements will occur only when patients and physicians come together to change the system.

As Abraham Lincoln said more than 150 years ago, "Public sentiment is everything. With public sentiment, nothing can fail. Without it, nothing can succeed."[2] The same holds true today. A revolution in primary care is needed; the public must demand a change. Through this book, I hope to encourage you to join in and push for the needed changes. It is critical to your health, your parents' and your children's health and your country's health. In these pages, I will show you what needs to be done and how to do it. Working together, you can create a *primary care system that offers high quality care to satisfied patients through enthusiastic and energized physicians at a reasonable price that lowers the total cost of care.*

PART I
BACK TO BASICS: PRIMARY CARE

We begin with an overview of what primary care is and is not and an explanation of the what and why of the primary care crisis followed by a look at true comprehensive primary care. Primary care as it should be is probably much more than you expect it to be or have experienced it to be. This is followed by a discussion of the healthcare paradox: despite outstanding biomedical science and excellent professionals, the American medical care *delivery system* is badly dysfunctional. We then explore the concept of integrative medicine, trust building and the all-important issue of healing.

CHAPTER ONE
THE PRIMARY PROBLEM WITH PRIMARY CARE

To understand the problem with primary care in this country, first consider this example of the value of a primary care physician. The PCP – the term I will use throughout the book for "primary care physician" – who was able to take the time needed to thoroughly listen to his patient and assess the situation.

One day, Dr. Gary Milles, a MDVIP retainer based physician who limits his practice to about 500 patients, saw Marsha, an enthusiastic and articulate patient he had known for many years. She came in for a minor problem, but he noticed that her speech patterns were slightly different from what he remembered in the past, so he spent considerable time conversing with her. No one who did not know her well nor anyone who had only a brief conversation with her would have recognized her speech had changed. The changes were subtle, but they were clear in Dr. Milles' mind. The rest of the medical history was unremarkable. He did a neurologic exam, which was also unremarkable, but he was certain that something was amiss. So he ordered an MRI of her brain. Her insurer refused to pay for it because she had no specific indications and an otherwise normal history and examination. Dr. Milles called the insurer multiple times to explain his rationale, and finally the insurer relented. The MRI showed a primary brain lymphoma – treatable, probably curable, because it had been caught early.

The message is simple. Marsha's PCP knew his patient well. Because he had an extended visit time with her, he was able to notice the subtle changes in her speech pattern. His skill, combined with a long history with his patient and adequate time, made all the difference and probably saved her life. Of course, it also illustrates another issue today – a serious problem with our current system of healthcare. In a legitimate effort to keep costs down, insurers routinely undermine the physician's autonomy to practice as he or she believes is best for patients.

To be effective, a PCP needs time to listen, diagnose, treat, prevent and – most importantly – think. Although short visits are fine for simple problems, they are not appropriate for someone who has multiple chronic illnesses and is taking five to seven prescription medications. And certainly not enough time for an elderly patient who may suffer from visual, hearing or memory problems nor for the person who presents with a problem that is somewhat out of the ordinary. In all of these situations, there is a tendency toward over-reliance on referrals to a specialist, which often means excessive testing and procedures. In many of these situations, all it takes is more time with the patient and primary care physician.

The term "primary care" refers to physicians who are in family medicine, general internal medicine and general pediatrics. Many obstetricians and some general surgeons serve, at least in part, as primary care physicians, especially in the latter parts of their careers. However, I will only refer to family medicine and general internal medicine doctors unless specifically mentioned to the contrary.

An Explanation of Comprehensive Primary Care

Some people think of primary care as going to the doctor with the flu, a sprained ankle, a urinary tract infection or some other minor problem – what is known in the medical community as episodic care. Some people think of the primary care physician as a source for referrals or the person to ask what specialist to see for a problem. In fact, primary care is both of these but also much more. First and foremost, it is about developing a close relationship between you and your doctor – *relationship medicine* is the essential ingredient for trust building and for true healing. It is about dealing with those unexpected but frequent, minor but annoying medical problems that pop up over the course of life. It is also about treating more serious problems – sometimes acute, like pneumonia – but more often serious chronic illnesses, such as heart failure, asthma, high blood pressure and diabetes. Effective primary care is about working to prevent these chronic diseases from occurring or to slow the progression of disease once it has occurred. It is also about maintaining wellness and health throughout life. In short, your PCP can handle about 90-95 percent of your healthcare and can do it effectively and cost efficiently. Your PCP needs more time with you to do it fully and thoroughly. In fact, data supports the notion that a well-functioning primary care-based delivery system not only increases quality of care but decreases costs compared to our current specialist-based system.

The Shortage

One problem in the primary care-based delivery system is that PCPs are becoming extinct. It's true. Not many medical students – only about 20 percent – choose primary care as their career path. And older PCPs are retiring early. Many others are closing their practices or seeking employment at the local hospital. Plus, rural and urban poor areas have always seen a shortage of primary care physicians. Today, only 30 percent of all physicians practice primary care (compared to about 70 percent in most other developed countries and about 70 percent in the United States 50 years ago), and this percentage is shrinking at a steady rate.

Estimates indicate that America, which today has about 210,000 primary care physicians in active practice, will need an additional 52,000 PCPs by 2025.[3] Good luck. This is based on growth of the population (requiring 33,000 added PCPs), the aging of the population (another 10,000) and the added number of individuals who will have health insurance as a result of the Affordable Care Act (another 8,000). In fact, the number needed is substantially higher. If you accept my premise – which I will detail later – that a primary care physician (or nurse practitioner or physician assistant) should care for only 500-1,000 individuals rather than the current typical 2,500 or more, then the need is truly much greater.

New Doctors

About 25,000 new graduates enter medical practice each year. With that, there are about 29 physicians for every 10,000 population, although they are not necessarily distributed evenly across all population areas or groups, for example, with fewer in rural and urban poor areas. Based on these numbers, one could argue that there is no shortage of doctors. Indeed, with the opening of new medical schools and many others increasing class sizes, there should be another 3,000 added to the graduating class each year, rising to 5,000 more by the end of the decade. But most graduates enter specialty care rather than primary care training, which means the ratio of PCPs to specialists will at best stay at 30 percent to 70 percent or, more likely, deteriorate further. Adding more specialists will only add to health care costs rather than increase quality.

Critical to how many PCPs are trained are two key factors. One is the paucity of trainee (or residency) slots available in the nation's teaching hospitals to train primary care physicians. Medical school graduates entering primary care take three years of post-graduate training, which includes an internship and two years of residency, often followed by an additional year or two in fields such as gerontology.

The key is that the vast majority of these residency positions are funded by the federal government via Medicare. Currently, Medicare pays teaching hospitals $9.5 billion each year to subsidize training for the next generation of physicians with residency programs that range from three to seven (or even more) years after medical school graduation. Medicare has kept these "slots" it will cover flat since 1997 and has given no indication of raising the number. But even more importantly are the absolute numbers of PCP vs. specialist slots available. There are simply many more specialist slots available. Medical centers want to train specialists. They represent assistance to the faculty or employed physicians, and they bring an aura of quality to the hospital. Any good professor – or chief of neurosurgery, for example – would want to have his or her own training program. It is a matter of pride. Absent a training program, the best will not choose to work for that medical center and will practice elsewhere. This is a serious conundrum for the medical center that needs the specialty program to drive more revenue. Additionally, although Medicare has been willing to pay for these specialty training programs over the years, it has not increased funding for primary care training.

A recent study[4] of 2006-2008 residency training and Medicare payments offers some interesting observations. Looking at the 20 hospitals that trained the most and the 20 that trained the least PCPs, respectively, among all teaching hospitals in the U.S., "the top primary care producing sites graduated 1,658 primary care graduates out of a total of 4,044 graduates (41 percent) and received $292.1 million in total Medicare graduate medical education (GME) payments. The bottom 20 graduated 684 primary care graduates out of a total of 10,937 graduates (6.3 percent) and received $842.4 million."[4] In other words, the hospitals that got the most money trained a larger proportion of specialists, which is logical if that is where the money is. However, in an era of serious primary care physician shortages, this makes little sense, especially since shortages will certainly worsen in coming years.

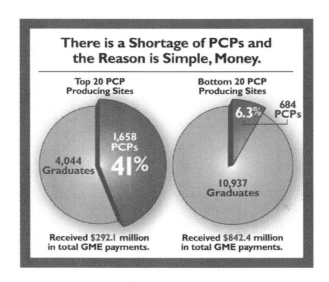

The PCP Position within Medicine

The other more critical problem is that primary care is not seen as a desirable career path today. The average PCP earns about $220,000 per year, according to a recent *New York Times* article.[5] A Medscape survey pegs it at $170,000 to $180,000 per year.[‡] That is in the range of what a first-year law school graduate earns if selected to join a large prestigious firm or what a first-year MBA graduate commands at a major consulting firm. It probably does not

---

‡ Most of the PCPs that I interviewed suggested that these income ranges are well above the averages that they are aware of from their own and colleagues practices.

seem like these PCPs are earning too little. It is a good income and certainly enough to keep the wolf from the door. Plus, most PCPs will tell you that they did not go into medicine for the money. They do it because they like people, solving problems, listening and doing good in the world. But – and this "but" is important – in inflation adjusted dollars, a PCP earns slightly less than what a PCP earned in 1970, yet sees twice as many patients per day to earn it.

In addition, primary care physicians earn about one-half of what a specialist earns. Specialists are generally seen to have a higher level of prestige in the community – "I was sent to Dr. Jones, *the surgeon*." Most medical school graduates have large debt loads (the current average is $170,000 with 40 percent owing more than $200,000), so earning more means paying it off sooner, and with a large debt, it is harder and scarier to take out a loan to start a practice that brings in fewer dollars. In addition, medical students realize that PCPs are in a non-sustainable business model, one which requires them to see far too many patients per day, accept unpleasant burdens with insurers, be on call many hours and yet not be able to offer what they know would be better care. In short, it is a practice on a treadmill with limited time per patient encounter and high levels of frustration. They see it as a no-win situation and so avoid primary care, even if that might otherwise be their preference.

The Money Question

In order to earn that $170,000-$220,000 income, PCPs must see too many patients each day and for too short a time to give the best possible care.

The system is based on what insurers pay for a visit. The office expenses must be paid first; what is left over goes to the physician. Given today's reimbursement environment, a PCP must see 25 or so patients per day to earn that $170,000-220,000. That means 15-minute visits with only 8-12 minutes of true "face time."

If PCPs cared for a reasonable number of patients and no longer saw 25 or more patients per day in their offices, then the PCP shortage would be much greater, perhaps by a factor of two to three or more. Yet when primary care physicians see fewer patients per day, they can then spend the time needed to listen, prevent, coordinate and think – four key activities that they often are not able to do effectively today. This means a need for substantially more PCPs.

So what's the solution? The fix is not to graduate more medical students but to make primary care desirable as a medical professional career. This means overcoming or changing the current non-sustainable business model so graduates, once again, choose to select primary care, thereby slowly but surely rebalancing the PCP-specialist ratio. This would, over time, greatly improve the delivery of healthcare.

Doctor's Thoughts and Another Patient's Story

I have published these thoughts on well-regarded healthcare sites, and these blogs often receive many comments and much debate. One doctor said, "Thanks, Dr. Schimpff, for your right-on diagnosis of our profession. Docs don't have the time to listen to patients, but even if they did, few know how to do it well. Skilled listening is useful for accurate diagnosing, but it can also treat emotional suffering. If we limit our work to simply diagnosing and treating physical illness in a rushed atmosphere, we're no longer physicians, but technicians working an assembly line."

Another commented: "I am an internist - I am a doctor. Go ahead - take away all the tests and imaging since the 1950s. Give me my light, my stethoscope, my mind and my hands. Give me enough time with my patient. I have diagnosed some pretty rare birds this way - onset of AIP, GBS, Crohn's. 'Dia-gnosis' from Greek means 'through-sight,' roughly. The patient encounter is the ONLY critical element in the practice of medicine, and the cheapest."

Another PCP, who had converted his practice to direct primary care, which I will explain as a new model later in this book, told me: "My utilization of hospitals, specialists and testing is way down. The insurers, rather than the patients, should pay us the retainers because we are saving them huge amounts of money – much more than the cost of the retainer."

I think they are all correct. How can we ignore the calls from doctors to reinvigorate the system and improve the primary care experience, both for doctors and patients?

Consider another patient story sent to me by a friend. It comes back to the values of listening and trust in the doctor-patient relationship:

"My mother's real-world story is mostly about a cardiologist but touches on the very problem you describe about PCPs in a brief but pointed way.

"I took my mother to the cardiologist this week. He was 45 minutes late seeing us but did spend a good amount of time with her, mostly listening, trying to figure out her medical issue. Once he thought he'd hit upon what was causing the problem and the solution (which happily, did not involve a drug or surgery but behavior modification), he said he'd call her internist who she has been seeing for many, many years to tell him about the discussion. My mother waved her hand dismissively and said, 'He doesn't know me.' The cardiologist looked surprised and a little confused, but I understood. My mother was saying that her internist had not spent time listening to her and getting to know her unique situation like this cardiologist had done.

"My usually non-compliant and defiant mother called me the morning after her appointment to report she had done what he recommended and would continue to do so.

"Behavior modification is not an easy prescription to give out, especially to the elderly. But his unhurried gentle questioning, sympathetic listening and obvious desire to figure out how to help her is what made my mother trust him. And although he kept us waiting for 45 minutes, when we left, I felt that my mother had actually consulted with a physician – a healer."

This story has both a good and not-so-good side. The good is obviously that the cardiologist listened to her and then developed a plan of action – with her and her daughter – that she could accept and follow. The not-so-good, or even unfortunate, is that she felt her PCP internist who she had visited for many years did not really know her, simply because he did not listen.

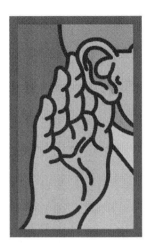

Here is another story on the importance of listening from Dr. Elias Anaissie, a specialist physician in an academic practice who was expected by his superiors to keep his patient visits short – about fifteen minutes. He wrote, "Many docs go along with the 'all inclusive – though unsafe – 15 minute visit.' Patients are very unhappy but they have no choice and end up paying with their health. This 'efficient' model actually leads to increased costs, worse outcomes and poor patient satisfaction. I recently saw a patient ... [who] had seen twenty doctors including seven during her three visits to [well known and respected clinic]. The specialists told her 'This is not cardiac,' 'not hematology,' not 'lungs,' etc. One of these specialists told her it was 'in her head.' She was desperate but she basically offered me her diagnosis during the 45 minutes I spent listening to her history. And since I do not type into the electronic health record ("the computer") during history taking, I was able to have a real connection with her – face to face. Her symptoms were very suggestive of dysautonomia and her 'Semitic nose,' just like mine, was consistent since as you know, this condition affects Ashkenazi Jews almost exclusively. The point is that looking at the patient and at not the computer gave me an additional - easily gotten - clue about her potential diagnosis...and today, most docs don't have the time to listen, to look at and/or observe the patients' demeanor let alone examine them. A strongly positive tilt table test confirmed the diagnosis. A good history with the doctor who saw her first would have saved her a year of agony and more than $500,000 in specialist visits and testing."

This lack of listening is the real care problem in American healthcare today. It is prevalent, pervasive and getting worse, not better. Listening takes *time*, but the PCP has too little time. Unfortunately, the electronic medical record, in many cases, accentuates this lack of listening as the doctor now focuses on entering data rather than maintaining eye, mental and emotional contact with you. But it is the inadequate income per patient in the current fee-for-service system that drives this lack of time and the lack of listening. Until the payment system is corrected and doctors have adequate time per patient to listen, healthcare will not be true care and certainly not healing.

Call this a future combination of *rights and responsibilities* – the doctor earns a decent income in return for offering superior care to a reasonable number of patients. This would be a good balance. But I venture to say that the "fix" will not be driven top-down but rather bottom-up. It will be when the PCP and the patient both decide that the status quo is no longer accept-able and they together reach a new arrangement in which the doctor can give high quality care, irrespective the insurance models.

The need is for a true "mind change" by patients and PCPs together. We need both patients and PCPs to take action and insist on change. This will require leadership to set out the aspirations, encourage others to join and then actually follow through with change. Perhaps this book can be part of the drive for that change.

Chapter Two

THE PARADOX IN AMERICAN HEALTHCARE

There is a real paradox in American healthcare. On the one hand, there are exceptionally well-educated and well-trained providers committed to our care. But, on the other hand, we have a very dysfunctional health care *delivery* system.

America is the envy of the world for its biomedical research prowess, funded largely by the National Institutes of Health and conducted across the county in universities and medical schools. The pharmaceutical and biotechnology industries continuously bring forth lifesaving and disease-altering medications. The medical device industry is incredibly innovative and entrepreneurial. The makers of diagnostic equipment such as CT scans and handheld ultrasounds are equally productive.

Consider these examples: The science of genomics is revolutionizing medical care in profound ways, such as producing targeted cancer drugs, predicting later onset of cardiac disease, offering prognostic data to guide cancer treatment, rapidly identifying bacteria and its antibiotic susceptibility, indicating whether a drug will work in a specific person and determining if a drug will cause a side effect in that person.

The pharmaceutical industry has brought us statins to reduce cholesterol, drugs to prevent blood clotting and effective means to control high blood pressure. The device industry has created a potpourri of new approaches that have transformed cardiac care, including angioplasty, stents, pacemakers and intra-cardiac defibrillators. We even have the ability to replace the aortic valve without major heart surgery.

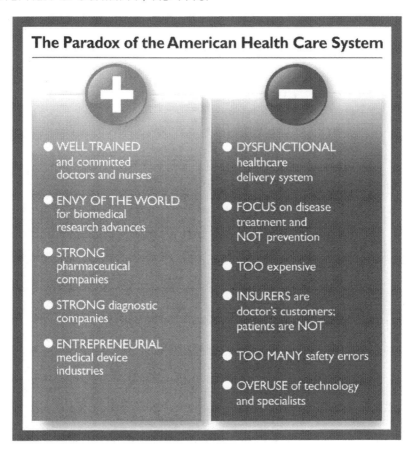

The Paradox of the American Health Care System

+

- WELL TRAINED
  and committed
  doctors and nurses

- ENVY OF THE WORLD
  for biomedical
  research advances

- STRONG
  pharmaceutical
  companies

- STRONG diagnostic
  companies

- ENTREPRENEURIAL
  medical device
  industries

−

- DYSFUNCTIONAL
  healthcare
  delivery system

- FOCUS on disease
  treatment and
  NOT prevention

- TOO expensive

- INSURERS are
  doctor's customers:
  patients are NOT

- TOO MANY safety errors

- OVERUSE of technology
  and specialists

Organs can be imaged noninvasively in incredible anatomic detail while also showing their inner cellular workings. The operating room is equipped with devices that make surgery less invasive, more effective and much safer. Simulation technology is completely changing how trainees learn the basics of procedures from the simple, such as drawing blood, to the complex, such as laparoscopic surgery. Robots are assisting surgeons in open heart and prostate surgery and are integral to today's large hospital pharmacies and central sterile supply systems.

The electronic medical record allows rapid access to information at any time and place, helps the physician to select the correct medication and dose and speeds up prescription transfer to the patient's local pharmacy. Radiology and pathology images can be sent via the Internet to a distant site for interpretation by a specific expert. A video of a surgical procedure can be evaluated by a distant authority to give advice to the operating surgeon, which is especially helpful in a battlefield situation far from home. And some surgery can even be done distantly via robotic controls.

We can be appropriately awed, proud and pleased about what is available for our care. But the care *delivery* system is highly flawed and dysfunctional. You can see this in many venues. America spends nearly 18 percent of its Gross Domestic Product on medical care, which is almost double that of the average of 9 percent for the other 34 economically-developed countries (such as Canada, Britain, France, Germany and Japan) in the Organization for Economic Cooperation and Development.[6] On a per capita basis, America spent $8,508 on health as of 2011, which is 2.5 times the $3,339 average of the other countries. Despite these expenditures, our lifespans are somewhat shorter. There are 100,000 preventable hospital deaths each year, and there are 100,000 deaths due to hospital-acquired infections. It is not an enviable record, and you get all of 15 minutes with your primary care doctor. Plus, these incredible technologies and lifesaving drugs are often used in ways or settings in which the marginal benefit barely, if at all, exceeds the marginal cost.

A report from the National Research Council and Institute of Medicine, summarized by the chairs in the *Journal of the American Medical Association*,[7] found "the health outcomes [of the United States] are generally worse than those of other wealthy nations. People in the United States experience higher rates of disease and injury and die earlier than people in other countries. Although this health disadvantage has been increasing for decades, its scale is only now becoming more apparent." Although there is better control of high blood pressure and cholesterol and there are lower cancer and stroke mortality rates, U.S. citizens have a lower life expectancy, higher infant mortality, higher rates of premature birth and thus lower birth weights, a higher incidence of HIV-AIDS, the highest prevalence of obesity and diabetes and the second highest rate of death from coronary artery disease, among other ills. Not an enviable record, especially for the level of expenditures.

Our current delivery system was designed during the past century with the expectation that the patient would pay the doctor a reasonable fee for the effort, skill and time involved. During the past 60 years, insurance developed initially to pay for the unexpected, highly expensive visits, such as surgery or hospitalization. Over time, insurance transitioned into what is essentially prepaid medical care, eliminating the financial "contract" between you and your PCP.

The delivery system developed to deal with *acute* medical problems, where it is reasonably effective. Consider the pneumonia that a single internist can treat with antibiotics, an appendicitis that can be cured by the surgeon or the fractured arm that can be cast by the orthopedist. But our medical care system works poorly for most *chronic* medical illnesses, and it costs far too much. Chronic illnesses include diseases like diabetes with complications, cancer, heart failure and chronic lung and kidney disease.

These chronic illnesses are increasing in frequency at a rapid rate. They are largely (although not entirely) preventable. A myriad of social, environment, financial and personal reasons have led to overeating, non-nutritious diets, lack of exercise, chronic stress, and smoking. Obesity is now a true epidemic, with one-third of Americans overweight and one-third obese. This results in high blood pressure, high cholesterol and elevated blood glucose, which combined with the long-term effects of the above behaviors, leads to diabetes, heart disease, stroke, chronic lung problems, kidney disease and cancer.

Once any of these chronic diseases develop, it persists for life, particularly diabetes and heart failure. These are complex diseases to manage and expensive to treat – an expense that continues for the rest of the person's life. Preventing them is equally complex but a lot less expensive. Good primary care can be a major stimulus to maintain wellness and avoid disease.

Although not properly appreciated, primary care physicians can handle most of today's chronic illness care. They have the knowledge, experience and skill level to do so. But this does not happen with short visits. All too frequently, the patient is referred to a specialist with the attendant increased costs of care, and the various specialists are not a true team working in a unified manner. Of course, many patients with chronic illnesses will need a team of caregivers. Consider a patient with lung cancer who may need a surgeon, radiation oncologist, medical oncologist, pulmonologist, pain specialist, palliative care team, nurse practitioner and many others. Primary care physicians generally do not spend the time needed to coordinate the care by the specialists of those with chronic illness, which is absolutely essential to ensure good quality at a reasonable cost. Any team needs a quarterback, and in general, that person is the primary care physician. The PCP needs to be the orchestrator as much as – if not more than – the intervener. This need for a team and a team quarterback for the patient with a chronic illness is much different than the needs of the patient with an acute illness in which one physician can usually suffice. This shift to a population that has an increasing frequency of chronic illnesses mandates a shift in how medical care is delivered. Unfortunately, our delivery system has not kept up with the need.

When the famous bank robber, Willie Sutton, was asked why he robbed banks, he replied, "That's where the money is." In healthcare, the money is in chronic illnesses. These consume about 75-85 percent of all dollars spent on medical care. So the need is to focus there. Adequate time with the patient with chronic illness and team development are key to the supply side of the problem. Developing patient engagement and self-care is the key to the demand side of the equation.

The place to start is with prevention. Since most chronic illnesses are preventable, we need aggressive preventive approaches, along with attention to maintaining and augmenting wellness. This would reduce the burden of disease over time and greatly reduce the rising cost of care. Unfortunately, America places far too few resources into wellness and preventive care, whether that is in regard to school lunches, employment wellness programs, insurance rebates for healthy living or many other possibilities. In addition, most providers (particularly primary care physicians) do not give high-level preventive care. They do screenings for high blood pressure, cholesterol and various cancers, and they attend to immunizations. But this is not enough. Patients need counseling on tobacco cessation, stress management, good eating habits and more exercise. They need an admonition to not drink and drive, not text and drive and to buckle up. They need to be reminded that dental hygiene today pays big dividends later in life. They need someone to listen closely to uncover the root cause of many complex symptoms. All of this takes time.

For the patient who already has a chronic illness and is sent for extra tests, imaging or specialists' visits, the expenditures go up exponentially, yet the quality does not rise commensurately. Indeed, quality often falls. Consider Henry's story.

Despite taking 23 – yes, almost two dozen! – prescription medications, Henry did not feel well. Plus, the expenses were beyond his means as a retiree, even with the help of his Medicare Part D drug coverage. Why so many medications? He had four different doctors, each writing prescriptions, often for the same diseases, but not in concert with each other. Once Henry got a primary care physician to coordinate his care, it was but a few months until he was down to seven medications. He began feeling much better, and he was saving himself (and his insurer) a substantial amount of money each month.

Henry was fortunate to find a primary care doctor who would devote the time needed to fully coordinate his care. But most primary care physicians find they do not have enough time for care coordination or for more than the basics of preventive care. And they do not have time to listen and think.

Henry's story points to another problem – clearly America has a *medical* care system and not a *health* care system. American medical care focuses on a disease once it has occurred but gives relatively little attention to maintaining health and wellness and proactively dealing with chronic illnesses once they develop.

Not only is the insurance system faulty, but many Americans do not have health insurance or are underinsured. As they obtain insurance or join the Medicaid ranks as the result of healthcare reform, there will be far too few primary care physicians to care for them. These individuals will, therefore, continue to use the emergency room as their primary place for care. Others who actually have a PCP will also use the ER when they think an issue needs resolution sooner than they think the PCP will see them. Alternatively, they will go to urgent care centers or the walk-in clinics being developed by chain pharmacies such as CVS, Walgreens and Wal-Mart.

Our system of care is not customer-focused. Doctors believe they have the patient's best interest in mind, but their work is not customer-focused as it is in most other professional-client relationships. You, as a patient, are not the customer of the physician. Since the insurer will determine whether and how much the physician will be paid for attending to your needs, you are largely a bystander in the relationship. The doctor's customer has become the insurer. You wait weeks and sometimes even months for an appointment – with the national average at 20.5 days – spend long times in the waiting room and are frustrated that you get only 10-12 minutes with your doctor. During this short appointment, your doctor interrupts you within 20 seconds and recommends you see a specialist, yet he does not personally call the specialist to explain the issue nor to smooth the path for a speedy appointment.

As for the insurers, you are likely not their customer either. Their customers are the ones who pay them – your employer or your government. It shows in our long waits on the phone and complex, hard-to-understand paperwork. It becomes apparent when you're frustrated that your insurance does not cover your latest tests, X-rays or specialist visits. Even those of you who purchase your own insurance as a self-employed or service industry worker do not find your insurer any more responsive than if your insurance came via an employer or the government.

So we are not the insurer's customer nor are we the doctor's customer. We are mere bystanders. This is hardly the type of contractual relationship you have with your lawyer, plumber, contractor or accountant. This urgently needs to change.

Who is to blame for the current state of affairs? Each party looks to the other, but perhaps each should hold up a mirror and take a closer look. Based on a recent survey, 90 percent of physicians say the medical system is on the wrong track. Beyond that, 83 percent are thinking about quitting, 85 percent think the patient-physician relationship is deteriorating, 72 percent do not think the Affordable Care Act individual mandate will lead to improved care, and 70 percent think the single best fix would be reducing government intrusion. Further, 49 percent will no longer accept Medicaid patients, and 74 percent are considering not accepting new Medicare patients. Finally, 80 percent believe doctors and other medical professionals are the ones most likely to help solve the mess.[8]

So the paradox is that America has the providers, the science, the drugs, the diagnostics and the devices needed for outstanding patient care. But there is a new type of disease – complex, chronic illness, mostly preventable, for which American medical care has not established good methods of prevention or adequate methods of care once developed. What should be the role of the primary care physician has been compromised by the insurance system, and all of this is exacerbated by an insurance industry that puts the incentives in the wrong places. The result is a sicker population, episodic care and expenses that are far greater than necessary

A new vision for our system must make it a *health* care, not just a *medical* care system. It must recognize the importance of intensive preventive care to maintain wellness and it must do so prospectively from the perspective of the population not just an individual who appears in the doctor's office. It must address the needs of those with chronic illnesses to both improve the quality of care and dramatically reduce the costs of care. It must be redesigned so the patient is the customer. Most critically, America needs many more primary care physicians (and other primary care providers) – the backbone of the healthcare system – who are able to offer outstanding preventive care, care for most illnesses, care coordination for chronic illnesses and testing procedures. They should do it in a manner that is satisfying to doctor and patient alike, with true healing and expert medical care. It is doable, but it means rethinking how our delivery system is structured and how PCPs are paid.

CHAPTER THREE
WHY PRIMARY CARE MATTERS

"As a hospital employed PCP, the system was to see more patients, do more, cut corners…it was not patient centered or patient-oriented as the hospital claimed in its marketing. That's baloney…they were only focused on the bottom line….I had a crackerjack office team but then the hospital merged three practices and dispersed the staff. The style I cared about for the front office was lost." Told to me by a physician who ultimately quit her hospital job and opened a retainer-based practice.

Your primary care physician needs to be efficient to see 25 or more patients per day and is likely frustrated with the circumstances. PCPs feel they have lost the autonomy to treat you as they perceive best for your health. Many are departing medicine or at least private practice. Primary care as we have known it for decades is rapidly transforming – and not always for the better.

PCPs need to address medical issues ranging from the very simple to the extremely complex. Many patients have multiple chronic conditions, take several prescription drugs, have various functional incapacities as a result of aging, and often have problems rooted in family dynamics or their own cultural norms and traditions. Good PCPs understand that the essence of care is the bond they develop over time with each patient. This relationship is the bedrock of the profession. But the current culture of medicine expects technology to be the answer, while financial requirements and legal concerns impose further burdens on PCPs. This combination has led to a fragmentation of care and the overuse of specialists and specialty care without coordination. Plus, technology is ubiquitous and trumps listening. Watch a medical TV show, and the doctors will use one technology after another – mostly because it is sexy. Listening is not. And unfortunately, the TV shows mirror medical school and residency training, which is another story entirely.

Today the PCP needs to be efficient. This means (sarcastically) that it is more efficient to give an antibiotic for a sore throat than to reassure the patient, and perhaps the parent, that it is likely caused by a virus. It takes more time to explain that the antibiotic will do no good and could even have undesirable side effects. It takes longer to explain that time is often the best medicine. And if reassurance is not done thoroughly, the patient likely will go away unhappy, assuming that he got "nothing." So PCPs sometimes do the quick action – give the antibiotic and add for good measure, "This should do it!" Although much can be done over the telephone or with email, which would prevent a trip to the office or even the ER, the efficient PCP wants to avoid both since there is no payment for either.

PCPs are frustrated. Some see the glass half full and many see it half empty. Those who see it half empty are quickly selling their practices to the local hospital or retiring early. Others are trying new payment methods. Traditionally, a newly minted physician would borrow funds to start a private practice or would enter an already established practice in town. In 2000, about 60 percent of physicians were in a private practice. This dropped to about 40 percent by 2012 and probably to 33 percent by 2013. It appears the decline in private practices is increasing with no end in sight. In 2000, about 20 percent of PCPs were employed by hospitals; today that number is up to about 40 percent and rapidly growing.

The question, of course, is why the rapid change? Some of it is related to the changing proclivities of the new generation of physicians. They have a desire for more personal and family time. They also want to better control their professional life, with a steady paycheck, fewer administrative obligations, and zero concerns about borrowing large sums to begin a practice. But this change to employed status is also about the current convoluted billing requirements of practice, the administrative complexity of running a business, and the ever-changing regulatory requirements.

We must acknowledge the tradeoffs, and the most important is autonomy – even outside of the private practice setting. Physicians have always valued their autonomy, but when they work for a corporation or hospital, no matter how benevolent, the company will have its own rules and regulations. The hospital might screen patients first for insurance coverage, whereas the private practitioner could decide who to accept. At a hospital, the PCP has little or no say in selecting nurses and other staff as coworkers. Autonomy is lost. Although the administrative burdens are fewer, physician are still expected to generate bills sufficient to cover salary and expenses. This means still seeing 25 patients or more to meet productivity standards. In this case, shifting to hospital employment does nothing to gain time to listen, prevent, coordinate and think.

The other tradeoff, although not directly relevant to the physician, is the increased cost of care with hospital employment. Often unwritten, the PCP is expected to meet certain performance targets of internal referrals. This includes the hospital's specialist pool and laboratory and imaging departments, even though it may mean a longer drive for the patient. In addition, the cost of an MRI is often much higher at the hospital than at a freestanding community radiology facility. As a patient, your out-of-pocket costs may not increase if you are well insured, but the total cost to the healthcare "system" increases greatly, as much as 2-4 times. This comes back to you in the form of higher premiums next year.

In this example, a pediatrician tries to understand the medical economics of a primary care practice.

"If we are going to make rational decisions about health care reform, it helps to understand the medical economics of a primary care practice. I was ten years out of medical school by the time I joined Narragansett Bay Pediatrics, a group practice in southern Rhode Island, and I was earning a salary of $48,000 for my part-time' position. I worked in the office 24 hours per week and covered nights and weekends. [A primary care pediatrician with ten years of experience working in a full time practice would probably have an income of about $125,000-150,000.] The hours on call were long and exhausting but generated very little income. The best way to make money as a pediatrician is to see as many outpatients with really good insurance as possible. Obviously, to see a lot of patients, you have to see them quickly. The easiest way to do that would be to give the parents exactly what they think they want – often antibiotics. That means writing the prescription for the over-priced broad-spectrum antibiotic before Mom has even settled into her chair, congratulating her for bringing her child in so soon.

"'That ear drum looked like it was about to burst!' Doctor to the rescue. It means treating any unexplained ache or fatigue as Lyme disease. 'Fortunately, we caught it so early.' 'Oh, thank you doctor,' gushes Mom, ushered out of the room six minutes after the doctor swooped in, relieved at the decisive action. A deeper conversation to tease out the vague symptoms and a recommendation for watchful waiting would have taken much longer, and, in all likelihood, a much less satisfied mom would be making her way to the check-out window.

"Quick patient turnover means telling stressed out nursing moms to switch to formula. 'You've done everything you could. Some women can't breastfeed. Let's get you a free sample case of formula.' What else is good for rapid patient turnover? Vitamins as the quick solution for a picky eater, cough syrup with codeine for colds and knee-jerk Ritalin for out-of-control kids. The child's condition will follow its natural course mostly unaffected by the intervention, and eroding reimbursement rates will be more than offset by the healthy volume of well-insured patients. On top of the financial disincentives to doing the job right, no one should underestimate the pressure pediatricians feel not to disappoint parents or how seductive it is for a pediatrician to be seen as coming to the rescue.

"Being conscientious has its price. 'This is a viral infection. You need to understand why antibiotics won't help, and may actually cause resistance,' or 'We have a lot of experience with Lyme disease here, and I don't think this is it. Why don't we follow this closely over the next few days? Call me if...' or 'Why don't you go ahead and breastfeed your baby now, so I can get a firsthand look at how he's doing,' or 'Insurance companies don't pay for....' Practicing good pediatrics is a moment-by-moment struggle. Most of the heroics in modern pediatrics are found not in the delivery room or the ER, but go unnoticed and unrewarded in the tiny little decisions of everyday care."[9]

This frenzied approach to practice, as described by this pediatrician, is leading to substantial "burnout" among PCPs. A national survey published in the *Archives of Internal Medicine* in 2012 reported that U.S. physicians suffer more burnout than other American workers, especially those in the "front lines" of care. Some 46 percent of physicians experienced at least one symptom of burnout: loss of enthusiasm for work, feelings of cynicism, and a low sense of personal accomplishment.[10] In a Medscape survey, internists were given a list of stressors and asked to rate how important they were as a cause of burnout. At the top of the list were factors that suggested an excessive workload and loss of control over the profession, without adequate compensation: "too many bureaucratic tasks," "spending too many hours at work," "feeling like a cog in a wheel" and "income not high enough."[11]

When doctors do not have enough time to really listen, the result is that they do not listen. A study of primary care physicians observed throughout patient visits revealed that the doctor interrupted the patient within 18 seconds on average.[12] "In only 23 percent of the visits was the patient provided the opportunity to complete his or her opening statement of concerns," which usually takes two minutes or less.[13] This is not only remarkable but a sad commentary on the short visit and the lack of attention by physicians to actually listen to the patient.

Doctors who make eye contact with their patients are perceived as spending more time than those who do not. This was discovered in a study in which all of the doctors were allowed a fixed amount of time in the exam room with the patient. The difference was about creating a connection with the patient.

PCP as CEO

Consider the PCP who has 2,500 patients. With the average American consuming nearly $8,000 of medical expenses per year, our hypothetical PCP is – or could be – directing the expenditure of nearly a total of $20,000,000. A sizable sum. Multiply that by all PCPs and it is quite sizable. PCPs cannot control how all of the dollars are spent, but when there is a good relationship with each patient, enough time with each and all care is coordinated, then the PCP is in a good position to direct how most of these dollars are spent. In this book, I advocate for a much smaller number of patients per doctor so there is time to give appropriate care. Let's assume 1,000 patients per doctor – that is still $8 million that he or she can be involved in managing. When primary care works at peak efficiency, costs come down substantially. People with serious chronic illnesses, such as diabetes or heart failure, consume substantial care requirements but even here the PCP can have a dramatic impact. Simply stated, relationship-based comprehensive primary care offers better care and, although it costs more for primary care, the result is not only better health but much reduced total costs of care.

Changing Nature of the Practice of Primary Care

During my interviews, nearly every PCP mentioned *first* that lack of time was the biggest issue – not enough time per patient to listen, coordinate care, discuss diet and exercise as part of thorough preventive care or to stop and think.

The time shortage is because of the need to meet overhead costs by seeing many patients per day. Overhead includes not only the receptionist, nurse and rent but also a full or part-time business person and accountant, a billing clerk or company, plus malpractice insurance, disability insurance and health-care insurance for all staff. This adds up to about $210,000 per year for one physician in private practice. Each visit brings, on average, about $65 from the insurers. To achieve a $150,000 income, this requires a total revenue of $360,000. That means 5,569 visits per year – or 22 per day – and about $27 per visit toward the PCP's income. Simply put, the PCP works until about 2 p.m. to cover overhead costs and then begins to accumulate dollars for his or her salary. See fewer patients and earn a lot less – remember, the office expenses still must be paid off first so the amount per visit to the PCP goes down fast if the number of patients seen per day is decreased. That is why a typical PCP sees so many patients per day and has 2,500 or more patients in total. That means 15-minute visits with only 8-12 minutes of true "face time."

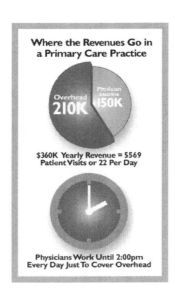

Where the Revenues Go in a Primary Care Practice

Overhead 210K | Physician Income 150K

$360K Yearly Revenue = 5569 Patient Visits or 22 Per Day

Physicians Work Until 2:00pm Every Day Just To Cover Overhead

Many PCPs feel they are "on the clock." Instead of maintaining a professional attitude, they begin to act, as one PCP said to me, like a "Home Depot mentality." Instead of high quality, the concept is to see how many patients they can fit in during one day. The root cause is the reimbursement system, in which Medicare – followed by commercial insurers – pay for primary care at low rates, thus driving the need to see too many patients per day. In addition, many PCP interview respondents said all of the Medicare rules and regulations, insurance company mandates, Medicare fraud dictums and malpractice litigation take up time that should be spent on the patient and tend to force physicians toward defensive medicine, which further increases costs.

Some PCPs observe what they feel is an ethical or professional change in newly minted PCPs (and all emerging doctors). Many do not put their patients first. They want time off, better on-call schedules, and more. A good family life is important, these experienced PCPs say, but the commitment to the patient is no longer paramount. They ascribe some of this change to the new residency rules, which limit on-call hours and foster a shift-work mentality, by which no one resident feels a full responsibility for the patient. It used to be "your problem" until it was resolved, but now the mindset is different. They can leave the problem for the next shift to sort out.

On top of that, new communication technologies such as email, Skype and social media are changing doctor-patient relationships and the ways practices will change for the future. Do these new approaches to interaction and communication help patients or further take away from patient time in the office? PCPs fall on both sides of the argument.

My interviews returned a wide range of usage related to email. Two physicians in retainer-based practices use email extensively, but they tell patients not to use it for acute problems since the PCPs may not look at their emails until late in the day or the next morning. For acute problems, they want the patient to call the office or cell phone. Email is handy for refills, answering general questions and making suggestions, they say. One physician noted that he can send an email to all of his patients at once about key issues, such as a notice that his office was flooded after a major water main ruptured. Other PCPs in more typical practices noted that the time they spend on emails is not compensated, and time is at a premium. Another family medicine physician said she uses email with her teens, and that has proven to be a good way to communicate with them. She tends not to use it with other patients, stating as others did, that she is not paid for emails. None reported using Skype with their patients.

Although habits are changing, doctors mostly do not use social media to engage patients. My interviews found a wide range of interests and usage. A few have Facebook pages for general information, but none invite their patients to be friends on their personal Facebook page. None that I interviewed are now using Twitter or YouTube. Healthcare lags behind other sectors in the use of social media, perhaps because it is a more conservative discipline or privacy issues. Like it or not, social media is here to stay and will become the "norm." As Kevin Pho, MD, founder of medicine's most widely-read blog and a primary care physician himself, points out, social media is where the patients are. Physicians need to be there also, or they will lose their influence.[14]

Entering Practice

Dr. Rebecca Crow wrote on KevinMD "As a graduating senior resident [i.e., she is in her third year of primary care residency] I'm scared to practice outpatient medicine. In a community of patients and physicians crying out for primary care doctors, what are we doing at a training level to foster and promote confidence and independence at doing this? I don't feel prepared and don't feel successful in that world. Who wants to pursue a career bought up in a sense of failure? Despite training at a community medicine outpatient minded program, I still feel more comfortable and successful in the inpatient setting. There has to be a better way to present clinic medicine to young doctors or there is no hope to reducing the primary care void using new physicians."[15]

After the rigors of medical school and residency, the time comes when the doctor steps out, becomes licensed and board certified and begins to practice medicine independently. Most PCPs that I interviewed say they were both elated and excited to finally begin their own practice, yet they also soon learned that they had more to learn. In interviews, respondents stated the four years of medical school and three years of residency training were not enough to feel like a well-functioning PCP at the outset. As a result, it takes two or three years to become comfortable practicing independently. Spending significant time in a practicing physician's office during residency helps, as does moonlighting in a clinic during the last year of residency, they say. Both of these experiences not only emphasize commonly seen issues in practice but also help a budding doctor to understand the mechanics of practicing medicine effectively and efficiently. Training programs are light in some areas, such as understanding patient costs for tests, procedures and drugs. "Training programs are just not designed to cover many of the non-medical basics that a new physician will encounter," one doctor told me. Among these are the business aspects of opening and managing a practice and understanding, from a business perspective, how the entire health care system operates. Many PCPs also recommend that trainees obtain some education in how to lead and communicate in a medical environment. "Leadership is not inborn but learned," another said. Other training that can be helpful to the PCP includes motivational interviewing, some understanding of public health and community health programs, and more training about the medical home model of care. They also said PCPs needed more time to understand complementary medicine practices, especially since their patients use many of these modalities with or without their PCPs' blessings.

Medical students, residents and newly emerged PCPs (and other physicians as well) often have little fundamental understanding of basic financial concepts. They have not had the time to focus here but, as in any profession, some training and education in personal and business finance is highly desirable, if not absolutely essential. Since it does not come with medical school or residency, it is up to the newly minted physician to find a trusted source of information and advice.

Mentors are critical during training. Most physicians who were interviewed felt there were few mentors in medical school or residency who actually spent time focused on deep listening and healing body, mind and spirit. That is probably because the professor also had too little time or was not attuned to that aspect of healthcare. Plus, medical schools rarely "honor" the professors for skills in these areas. It does not lead to promotion.

My own observations from medical school, residency and more than 40 years in an academic medicine setting are that far too little time and attention is paid to the "art" of medicine. Most training is directed at the technical, the diagnostic or therapeutic procedure, and too little is spent on actually listening to the patient and becoming truly aware of the patient's anxieties, family and life situations and other factors that uniquely affect the medical situation. More effective mentoring is definitely needed.

A PCP educator/clinician suggested that many of the best trainees in primary care are those who have had a broad humanities background before medical school and who have shown some proclivity toward service to mankind while in high school and college. He felt that these were the types of individuals who could most effectively become good primary care physicians because their background of service and broad education served them well.

No matter what was learned in training, medicine is a lifelong learning experience, so the PCP needs to develop a method to stay abreast of new findings. The need is to stay current, and the challenge is to find time to do so.

Primary care is a difficult, complex specialty to practice. It takes years of training and additional special skills. The current environment is discouraging students from choosing primary care as a career and accelerating the migration from private practice. A growing population of PCPs is critical to a successful healthcare system. Without a strong foundation of primary care physicians, our healthcare system will crumble, while costs – physical, emotional and monetary – continue to rise.

Chapter Four
BRINGING BACK THE HUMAN SIDE OF HEALING

All physicians perform well in college, score well on the Medical College Aptitude Test and interview well during the admissions process. Then they spend four years in medical school and a minimum of three years in residency training. Some choose primary care, and others choose a specialty for their careers. Do certain characteristics distinguish the primary care physician from the specialist? And do particular characteristics set some PCPs above the rest?

Who Becomes a Primary Care Physician?

Ask PCPs, as I have with these in-depth interviews, and they will tell you that certain types of individuals are drawn to primary care careers. As a general rule, PCPs like people. This was true of them long before they started medical school, and it only blossomed further during training. They like to talk to people. They enjoy getting to know a person – their ideals, goals, ambitions, cares and sorrows. They are interested in learning from the patient rather than talking down to the patient. Their ego can be strong, but not to impose themselves on the patient. They tend to want to know their patients and understand their place in family and society. PCPs want to know the "whole story," and they tend to see the patient as a whole person, as part of a family and a community. They see the patient as a unique individual and the illness as part of that totality of the person, not only a diseased organ or system. PCPs generally like to engage in an intellectual puzzle and like to solve a mystery. They have a "general contractor" mentality, meaning they see themselves as capable of getting most of the job done themselves. However, they are also comfortable drawing in others and are committed (if not always able due to time constraints) to coordinating everyone involved in the patient's care. This makes them the "captain of the ship," or the integrator of everyone involved. Although PCPs wish to earn a good income, money is not the most important aspect of their lives nor is it what drove them to become physicians.

Characteristics of a Good Primary Care Physician

Richard Belitsky, MD, the deputy dean for education at Yale Medical School, talked to the freshman class a few years ago at their White Coat Ceremony.[16] In part, he told them there was much to learn "but so much of what you need to be really good doctors, you already know… Becoming a great doctor begins not with what you know, but who you are. Being someone's doctor is about a relationship. That relationship is built on trust… Being a great doctor begins not with what you have to say, but your ability to listen."[17]

A patient, Samantha, told me about a medical experience that was the opposite of what Dr. Belitsky advised his doctors-to-be.

"I've had unsatisfying and frustrating experiences with a doctor lately. Beginning six months ago, I've had increasing GI pain and discomfort. Four months ago, the pain and discomfort had increased so much I made a doctor's appointment. She [the doctor] entered the room looking bored and she gave me the feeling she had something better to do. I was asked a lot of questions, and she made a lot of notes but she never *talked* to me! It was not a conversation. She suggested the problem was reflux. I told her I had a lot of experience with reflux and that whatever was going on didn't feel like that. I pointed to the area and said, 'I can outline for you exactly where my pain is.' No response. I tried to engage her in conversation, but her responses to me were pretty much one sentence, and to say more than 'yes' or 'no' seemed an effort. I told her all of my symptoms and what I had been doing to alleviate them. It was like talking to a robot.

"I did not respond to her treatment prescription, and so eventually she sent me for an upper endoscopy. As I expected, my esophagus looked totally normal; what I did have was gastritis. I looked up the symptoms of gastritis and there it was – I had a textbook case. Why had she not discussed the possibility with me? Did she not consider it a possibility? Yes, I have a reflux history, but why treat me for reflux when my symptoms didn't fit that pro-file? It's what you said about the patient giving the doctor the diagnosis. If someone had stopped to really listen to me, costs could have been mitigated for the insurance company and for me. Maybe the endoscopy could have been avoided if anyone had taken the time to talk to me appropriately. Most importantly, I could have felt better sooner.

"One more thing, when I told my boss about the results of the endos-copy he said, 'Uh-oh, too much stress at work?' I know now that stress can be a major factor in gastritis, and yet the doctor only asked about my stress in a very perfunctory way, as if she just needed to check it off the list. Ask about stress – check the box – move on.

"Yet another frustrating, disappointing and expensive interaction with the medical community."

You may have had the same experience as Samantha. That is unfortunate but all too common.

Views From Practicing Primary Care Physicians

Primary care physicians report that listening is the key and most important attribute of being a good physician in primary care. By "listening," they mean one who listens to the patient's story without rushing it and without embellishing it. They allow the patient to develop his or her own story of the situation, perhaps with some prompts to help the focus but without unduly narrowing the narrative. Secondly, the PCP must be nonjudgmental if he or she wants to learn from the patient and develop a strong doctor-patient relationship. This strong relationship is the third major attribute. In addition, PCPs need to like people and like their patients. Good PCPs are well-grounded in basic medical science and the latest in evidence-based care and constantly seek continuing education. Good PCPs are also conservative, meaning they work with lifestyle, behaviors, nutrition and exercise before resorting to drugs or procedures. This requires patience; not everything can be "fixed" immediately.

Another important attribute is an innate sense of kindness and the ability to show kindness, even when rushed or stressed. They also have the ability to accept inconvenience (after hours phone calls, for example) and tolerance of others' missteps (when patients forget what pills to take and when). They feel that knowing the patient over the long term aids the care process and enhances the doctor-patient relationship, as does being attuned to the patient's physical, emotional and spiritual needs. Knowing the patient's family also helps to understand the patient, and the family can be the physician's ally. Combined, these develop the triad of trust, respect and partnership. As expressed by one PCP, "I need to be available, able and affable." In addition, the doctor must be a good role model, which means attending to personal weight, exercise, stress, smoking, health promotion and wellness. Some will not only be good physicians but also true healers, a desired state that only some attain.

Views From Interested Observers

When asked what constitutes a good doctor, the answers vary, but some of the most noted common attributes are these: Listener, commitment, compassion, humanity, attentive, patient, competent, teacher, healer and ethical. A good overview from one individual was, "I've met many a physician in 36 years of service. Some brilliant, some not so much. The one thing I have noticed about those who were great, truly great, were those who were humble but confident. They would listen quietly to a patient's story and were never really rushed nor found themselves panicking in a critical situation. They were stoic yet responsive and treated nurses, technicians and even field medics as a valued part of the team. To sum it up, they know who they are and where they came from. And like all of us, still put their trousers on one leg at a time. There really isn't a single word to describe greatness, it's part of the diverse nature of who they are and how they apply what they've learned and what they know."[18]

The Physician Scientist

The good physician, in any specialty, must have a superb grounding in biomedical science. That is why the first two years of medical school focus so heavily on the basics of anatomy, biochemistry, molecular biology, genomics, physiology, pathology, immunology, microbiology and pharmacology. Then come the years of learning the elements of diagnosis and treatment, initially during the latter years of medical school and then during internship and residency. It takes these initial years of education – but then a lifetime of continuous learning – because the science is always being updated and exponentially so. Continuing medical education is essential for a good physician as approaches to treatment and diagnosis improve at a rapid rate. Of course, doing this takes time, which is that key element in short supply.

The Integrative Medicine Physician

Beginning with a deep understanding of medical science and years of training and experience, the primary care physician also needs to know when it is important – or even critical – to call upon others with specific knowledge, techniques or approaches that might be best suited for a particular patient. Sometimes this means calling in the cardiologist, surgeon, gastroenterologist or psychiatrist. But it may also mean making good use of other modalities and practitioners, such as chiropractic, social work, acupuncture, psychology, massage, nutritional therapy and exercise physiology.

Integrative medicine means a healing environment and a passion for prevention and wellness in addition to diagnosis and treatment. It also requires working with the patient and the patient's family as partners, understanding the deeper causes of illness and symptoms, providing approaches for self-care, and taking enough time to address all of the patient's concerns. For some integrative medicine physicians, it also means being intimately familiar with proven complementary practices, such as acupuncture, yoga, massage, nutrition coaching and personal fitness training. Some PCPs have learned techniques such as meditation or the Benson relaxation response and can use or teach their patients directly.

But at its core, integrative medicine means a strong relationship between patient and doctor, a relationship that is a partnership, one that deals [not only] with medical issues but also those factors that can contribute to reduced wellness and loss of health, such as poor nutrition and lack of exercise. It means addressing stress, spirituality and in general an expanded sense of connectivity between doctor and patient.

For example, this patient story about an integrated approach to a medical dilemma comes from Delia Chiaramonte, MD, director of education at the University of Maryland Center for Integrative Medicine, who is board certified in Family Medicine.

A medical student had suffered from severe headaches for many years that limited his quality of life and effectiveness as a student. His personal physician identified them as cluster headaches a few years before and tried standard medications without much success. Dr. Chiaramonte evaluated him differently using an integrative approach. She listened intently as he talked about his headaches, lifestyle, diet, physical activity, stress and school work. Like almost all medical students, he studied hard. He said he stayed up until about 3 a.m. studying, many times because he could not fall asleep earlier. His diet included doughnuts and other high carbohydrate and processed foods, plus about twelve cups of caffeinated coffee each day, sometimes interspersed with colas. He had no time for exercise. He sat – hunched over – in front of his computer for many hours each day, and his posture showed it.

Instead of recommending other diagnostic procedures or new medications, his integrative medicine "prescription" included the following: He needed to start a better diet that included protein at breakfast and healthy snacks during the day, and he needed to establish a set time for exercise. He should get away from the computer for 10 minutes every hour and walk around and stretch. He should also get eight hours of sleep each night and go to bed by 11 p.m. To assist him with this plan, he was scheduled to see a nutritionist to devise a more healthy diet. He also needed to work with a personal trainer to establish the exercise program – one that could be done anywhere without impacting his studies. In addition, she recommended that he visit a chiropractor to release his sternocleidomastoid muscles and other neck muscles back to their normal length. Since caffeine has a long half-life in the body, he should stop drinking caffeine after noon each day. The combination of a better diet, exercise and less caffeine meant he should be able to study more effectively and sleep better.

Given the pain and debility of his headaches, he was more than willing to give this prescription a try, though he was somewhat skeptical since it included no medication. But it worked. The headaches disappeared, he felt generally better, he was no longer drowsy in class and he began to truly enjoy medical school. And he did not need to take any medication.

This is the power of integrative medicine. It used a holistic approach that began with careful listening and then brought to bear many different disciplines, including the best of Western scientific medicine plus nutritional medicine, exercise physiology, stress management and chiropractic expertise. When used together and coordinated by one PCP, the combined approach had a dramatic effect.

The term "integrative medicine" is too often confused with unproven techniques that are used without seeking competent medical care. But many approaches have been in use for millennia and have been subjected to the tests of time. In recent years, many first-rate investigations have evaluated acupuncture, massage, meditation and various herbal remedies. Acupuncture, for example, has proven useful for many types of chronic and acute pain and for reducing the nausea of cancer chemotherapy.

Today, most medical schools teach about the proven complementary modalities, and some PCPs learn not only when to refer to them but also how to personally use some of these approaches. In my interviews, some PCPs – but certainly not all – were positive about complementary medicine. They felt it had real value, noted that most patients sought complementary practitioners anyway, and said there was increasing evidence-based data about the value of some techniques and practices. One PCP took a course in acupuncture for physicians and used it frequently. Another said, "I am very respectful of complementary medicine. I refer to chiropractic and many other complementary practitioners, just as I refer to behavioral health or surgery. I am learning every day. Patients are thirsty for complementary medicine. Traditional medical docs who are not on board are just behind the times." Yet another said, "Integrative medicine is not a catch-all for complementary medicine, it is just good primary care. I think of it as connoting the medical home concept. It is part and parcel of my practice." But many doctors, mostly those in practice for a longer period of time, said their knowledge was limited, and it was difficult for them to refer to complementary medicine practitioners. However, they responded to other questions that they frequently referred to nutrition, health and fitness coaches.

Most importantly, the PCPs all stated that the key attribute of the superb PCP (or any physician) is to listen – to listen deeply and without interruption as the patient explains the narrative of the situation. Such was the case with the medical student evaluation described above. In his case, it was about the totality of his life and how the headaches fit into that life story. Armed with that knowledge, his integrative medicine physician was able to offer ways to deal with the headaches through the root causes – an unhealthy lifestyle that dramatically affected his entire life and his ability to be an effective medical student.

Trust and the Physician

As a patient, you have probably had the experience of meeting a physician for the first time and quickly realizing that he or she has your best interests in mind. The feeling comes quickly; you become comfortable and less anxious. Unfortunately, you may have had the opposite experience of encountering a well-educated, well-trained physician who, although technically an expert, left you cold.

As a patient, have you ever thought that the doctor wasn't listening to you? Or did not seem to understand what was important to you? Was he talking in jargon but not in a language you could understand? Did she give you bad news and leave you hanging about what to do next? Unfortunately, these are the characteristics of the doctor who may be an expert but not engaged in true healing.

"The image of a patient and a doctor sitting knee to knee and heart to heart has come to look as quaint as a Norman Rockwell painting." This is a quote from The Bedside Manifesto by Dr. Jeff Kane.[19] Unfortunate but true.

That comfort, or the feeling that a doctor is "good" as a clinician, comes quickly because he or she creates a personal connection. Yes, PCPs must be knowledgeable. That is exemplified by the diplomas and certificates proudly framed on the office wall. However, it is that ability to "connect" that is part of the art of medicine. That is the added ingredient that makes the well-trained caregiver a true physician, nurse or other provider. Of course, it is also true that a physician with the "art" but no "science" is just a pleasant quack. What is it that gives you the sense of trust? More than anything, it is a physician who actually listens to you. He or she makes eye contact, maintains it, and does not turn around to use the computer to enter your history. You get full attention, and the doctor is nonjudgmental while validating your feelings and concerns. You get the sense that the doctor is telling you the truth, even when it is a message you would prefer not to hear. And your questions are answered in a way that you can understand, not in "medical speak." These are all attributes you pick up in the first few minutes while in the exam room or hospital bed. Over time, they educate you, lowering the huge information gradient between the two of you. That is when trust develops.

Another patient story illustrates how important listening is to trust and effective medicine.

"My mother [an elderly lady with many chronic illnesses] called me at work hysterical because the new 'pain' doctor had told her to call to let him know if the injection he'd given a week previously had worked for her lower back pain. She called to tell him that it had not, and during that call, she proceeded to describe to him some increase in her urinary issues. The doctor said there was nothing he could do for her and she needed to get to the ER for a work-up. I asked my mother, 'What does he want worked up? We can't take you into an ER and say "Work her up." They'll say, "Where should we start? She's a mess of problems!" ' She didn't really understand why she had been told to go, so I called the doctor. To his credit, he did speak with me for about five minutes and during the conversation said, 'I will admit that I have a hard time figuring out with your mother what is chronic and what is acute. But I am concerned that she may have a urinary tract infection.' The doctor said that if we chose to take her to her PCP for a urinalysis and evaluation that would be okay as long as she could be seen that day. He said, 'I leave it to your family's discretion.' She doesn't really trust her primary care physician because he 'never listens to me;' she felt she would get faster, better service at the ER. So we went there and they found a UTI."

A few observations: The pain doctor did appreciate that there was a problem, but other than saying "go to the ER," did nothing. The mother was older and did not fully understand his concern. He could have asked for her daughter to contact him or could have called her directly, but he did not. He also could have called her PCP directly, explained his concern, and asked that she be seen promptly, but he did not. Basically, he left a confused patient with a potentially serious problem in limbo. As for the PCP, the patient does not trust him because he does not listen to her, so unfortunately, she felt the ER was the better place to go. This adds to up a huge waste of time, people and money – in Medicare, Medigap and her own dollars – when the PCP, were he trusted, could have diagnosed and treated her quickly, effectively and inexpensively.

Doctors also need to listen – and probe, if necessary – to understand what underlying issues may have precipitated today's visit. Consider this analogy to the doctor visit: If you were driving your car and the "check engine" light came on, you would probably take the car to the garage for a checkup. What would you think if the mechanic only took out the little red light but did nothing else? In medicine, that is equivalent to learning about a patient's symptom, such as acid reflux, and simply treating it with an acid blocker like Nexium. The drug is good and may resolve the discomfort, but it ignores the underlying reason for the discomfort. Is it related to a chronic stressful situation at work or home? Is it a response to gluten sensitivity? Is it caused by an anatomic problem with the junction between the stomach and esophagus? Or is it an ulcer? Treating the symptom is not enough. It is important to get to the root cause.

A geriatrician told me about an episode when he ordered a blood count to check his patient for possible anemia. He promised to call the patient once the results were back later that day. The results came back that evening, but he was engrossed in various activities and never got to it. The next morning, he noticed the results on his desk, saw that it was normal, and continued with his rather hectic schedule. He planned to call the patient whenever he had some time. Later in the day, he found an email from the patient. It read: "I like you and think you are a competent doctor and I know that you are very busy. But you *failed* [my italics] me just now by not getting back promptly to me with the results of my blood test." The doctor, who prided himself on his caring manner and responsiveness, was deeply troubled and touched by the message. It was an important personal wakeup call. Although it happened some years ago, it is still uppermost in his mind today as he thinks about what patients really need from their doctors. They need to be able to trust, but it is hard to make and maintain trust when there is so little time.

Your primary care doctor must be well-versed in medical science and also the traits that define him or her as a physician you can trust. Medical advances, such as new drugs, imaging devices and operating room technology, are greatly expanding what can be done for patients. But concurrently, it seems that medicine is so technologically focused that the age-old art of being a healer has become a legend. What your doctor needs to remember is that you are a human with the needs of a human; the doctor needs humanism. Humanism in medicine can be summarized as a provider who likes people and listens deeply to them without being judgmental. Add to these the traits that exemplify the true healer.

Chapter Five

NOT ALL ILLS CAN BE CURED WITH A PILL: THE DOCTOR AS A HEALER

Healing is so important in medicine that it deserves a deeper discussion. There is a difference between being a modern day physician and being a healer. All societies have healers – wise men and women, shamans, medicine men and others. The "old time practitioner," like my grandfather, was almost always a healer, but many physicians today are not. It is an issue of interest, training, time and prioritization. Most individuals who aspire to be physicians probably aspire to be healers. But it requires training to be a healer just as much as it takes training to learn how to do an examination or an endoscopy. It requires good mentors, but they seem to be in short supply in most medical schools, and the standard post graduate training programs or residencies seem to "train out" rather than "train in" the healing skills.

Healing means to make whole or re-establish harmony and wholeness. It comes from the same root as holiness – a connection infrequently recalled in today's medical practice. The healer is the guide in the process. He or she can be a healer without necessarily curing a disease. A good doctor tends to the person who has a disease rather than just the disease itself, paraphrasing Sir William Osler, chief of medicine at Johns Hopkins Hospital at its inception in 1889 and known for his textbook of medicine. And as Dr. Kane puts it, "In our secular society, physicanhood was as close as one could get to a sacred calling."[18]

A report in the *Annals of Internal Medicine* suggested eight characteristics of the physician healer: He or she does the little things like make eye contact with you; takes time and listens to you; is open; finds something to like or love in each patient; removes barriers and does not sit behind a desk; lets you explain your illness; shares authority and remembers you are ultimately in charge; and is committed and trustworthy in your eyes.[20] One can be a physician yet not a healer, and not all healers need to be physicians. For example, a mother's kiss "heals" a child while the child's body slowly resolves the skinned knee. Many complementary medicine practitioners have the attributes of the healer.

Think back to the story of Susan in the Preface. She was referred to several specialists and offered multiple tests, procedures and surgeries, yet none of these physicians took the time to understand the underlying issue. Each was competent in the field, but each left her in limbo, never focusing on what brought her to medical attention in the first place. No one was a healer for her.

Dr. Mimi Guarneri, in her book *The Heart Speaks,* recalls the teaching of one of her professors. He was elderly [or so it seemed to the young residents], seemed to take forever talking to each patient, and was not to be rushed. The residents were frustrated that he "wasted" time. At the end of rounds one day, he said that he wanted to teach the residents and students something that they would otherwise never learn during their training. He said that it was important to "let your patients tell their stories, and if you really listen, they will give you the diagnosis. If you don't listen, you will miss the answer that is right in front of you."[21]

Her professor's point was that a symptom is often a "downstream" manifestation of a body's unconscious crying out for help. As described by Upledger in *Healers on Healing,*[22] a hemorrhoid may not be just a hemorrhoid. It may be a manifestation of liver cirrhosis, which is the result of years of alcohol excess, which in turn is the product of unresolved psychological issues. A careful history may illicit that guilt persisting from long ago – yet hidden from the patient's consciousness – has been the cause of the alcohol abuse. Helping the patient with self-discovery of the underlying guilt and working through it is true healing. It may result in less alcohol abuse, but the cirrhosis may nevertheless be permanent. The point is that merely sending the patient for surgical removal of the hemorrhoids, appropriate as that might be, misses the real illness and the opportunity to heal. Of course, the physician needs to be a careful listener and nonjudgmental in order to be effective. Recall that my in-depth interviews with primary care physicians consistently reported that being a good primary care physician requires one to be non-judgmental and a good listener. And, of course, that takes time.

The message is that nearly all diseases occur in a patient who has a narrative to offer. The PCP's role – if he or she desires to be a healer – is to listen to that narrative and uncover the deeper issues. Once found, these may be not only a surprise to the physician but to the patient as well. More often than not, "healing" is directed at the underlying psyche of the patient. The patient can then involve his "inner healer" to affect the needed changes. Thus, the really good doctor appreciates not only the anatomic and physiologic but also the underlying emotional or psychologic implications of a disease.

Years ago while in oncology training, I was on night duty when a patient of one of my colleagues had severe penile pain. Arthur had received a new investigational chemotherapy, and it turned out to have an unexpected effect of damaging the lining of the bladder and urethra. It gave him a strong uncontrollable urge to urinate, yet each time the burning was excruciating. Oral pain killers did not help and Pyridium, used for the burning of a typical urinary tract infection, was ineffective. Eventually, I found an anesthetic gel to squeeze into his urethra, which offered some relief – enough that he could sleep. My job for the evening was done. But I later learned that this pain had a much deeper meaning for Arthur. He had developed a close rapport with a long-time evening shift nurse. She told me that in college his classmate girlfriend became pregnant; she gave birth to the child, but he abandoned them. Now nearly a decade later, married to another woman and with two children, he had developed testicular cancer. That diagnosis plus tonight's pain was, he believed, God's punishment, and he was wracked with guilt. Arthur's oncologist never learned this because he only focused on the cancer itself. The nurse, who sat quietly and nonjudgmentally with the patient in the evenings, was the one who learned about his inner turmoil.

It is necessary to look within to find the root cause of discomfort. The disease may be a random event, but it may also be a manifestation of an underlying issue or, as with this patient, a new reminder of an old guilt. Treating the disease, even successfully, will not heal the underlying issue, and it will ultimately re-manifest itself as a recurrence or new symptom. Deep, nonjudgmental listening is the essential first step in healing. From there begins the therapeutic exchange. The nurse listened but did not judge, and as a result, that patient was able to open his heart to her.

Patient satisfaction surveys completed after hospitalizations are quite consistent. The patients may not love the food or parking arrangements, but they are deeply troubled that their doctor or nurse "didn't listen to me." Studies have shown that doctors tend to interrupt patients within seconds – not minutes – of them beginning to explain their illness. This is incredibly frustrating to the patient, and it means the real narrative is lost.

As the daughter of a patient told me, "This happened to my father repeatedly during his hospitalizations. It made him very angry although he was a very mild-mannered man. It bothered me and my siblings as well. I see it with my mother too because she can't always find the right words and I can palpably feel a doctor's impatience and so can my mother and it makes her communication worse."

Sometimes doctors do not even listen to their patients who are doctors themselves. I was once referred to an otolaryngologist (ear, nose and throat or ENT) doctor. I knew what I wanted to tell him, but it was obvious that he had already developed a diagnosis in his own mind within less than a minute of my arrival. I decided to politely insist that he hear me out, which he did, but I could sense it was with reluctance. He then did an exam and announced his original diagnosis was correct. A few weeks later, when his prescription did not create any improvement, he finally began to listen. He considered another diagnosis – one that was fairly obvious if he had listened the first time – and I finally received the proper treatment plan.

Consider another example of a medical school professor and general internist who learned the value of deep listening early in his training. As a resident in the primary care clinic, he had a patient who always ended up in the hospital. She did not seem to have any serious underlying diseases, and he thought he gave her good medical care. Still, she bounced into the hospital frequently. At one clinic visit, his attending faculty physician stepped in. She quickly developed a close rapport with the patient, delved deeply, and learned the woman needed someone to listen to her issues. No one was doing so, and her admissions to the hospital were her way of crying out for help and understanding. Armed with this new insight, the resident met with the patient regularly and listened in an empathetic and nonjudgmental manner, sometimes for 30 minutes, occasionally for more. The patient would pour out her heart to him. Later in practice in a community hospital and then at the university, he continued to care for her, mostly listening carefully in a nonjudgmental manner over a period of about 20 years. There were no more hospitalizations. Then came managed care. Her insurance mandated that she go elsewhere for primary care. The university overheads were too much for the managed care operator to tolerate. In less than a year, she was back in the hospital several times. The insurer saved money on primary care but paid the price in hospitalization bills. More importantly, a patient who could be helped easily with humane attention was no longer benefiting.

To quote again from Dr. Kane, "Sir William Osler said, 'the practice of medicine is an art, not a trade; a calling, not a business; a calling in which your heart will be exercised equally with your head. Often the best part of your work will have nothing to do with powders or potions.' Osler was disappointed that his warnings about science eclipsing art went unaddressed. When he left Johns Hopkins in 1904 for Oxford University he wrote to a colleague he considered too laboratory oriented, 'Now I go, and you can have your own way.'"[18]

Tolstoy wrote these three questions/answers, which the physician should keep in mind in order to be a healer:

> "What is the most important time?
> Now, no other time matters.
> Who is the most important person?
> The one you are with.
> What is the most important thing to do?
> To do good for that person."[23]

The physician who focuses on the patient, not just the disease, and who constantly respects the answers to these three questions can hope to aspire to be a healer. This healer is one who focuses solely on the patient with all of his or her senses and pays attention to body language, word use, metaphors – all to deeply understand and engage with the patient.

It is not only primary care physicians who are healers. Thomas Scalea, MD, is professor and director of the R Adams Cowley Shock Trauma Center at the University of Maryland Medical Center in Baltimore. The Shock Trauma Center is arguably the best trauma center in the country, if not the world. It admits only those 3-5 percent of trauma patients with the most extensive injury, yet survival consistently exceeds 95-97 percent. Credit this to Maryland's emergency transportation system, the Shock Trauma Center's exquisite teamwork, the well-trained staff and the best technology. The Shock Trauma Center might be the zenith of technologic prowess.

Dr. Scalea notes that despite all the sophisticated technology and surgical skills of the staff, the patient still needs the provider to be humanistic. For example, when he enters the room, he (and he encourages his staff to do the same) sits down to talk with the patient eyeball to eyeball at the same level, rather than the usual practice of standing as an imposing figure and looking down at the patient. He points out that the doctor (or nurse or other provider) needs to converse with the patient in clear English, not in medical speak. Medical speak is for the provider's convenience, but with a patient it leads to non-communication. As he puts it, the provider must "expect to repeat what he or she said today again tomorrow and again the next day; expect that the patient needs to hear it repeatedly. And the doctor should not be annoyed that the patient forgot it all by tomorrow morning."

When doctors visit a patient, it is important to listen. Listen hard and long. Dr. Scalea described a trainee who would stand behind him by the bedside and look across his shoulder at the patient. Somewhat annoyed by this intrusion into his "space," Dr. Scalea asked why the resident stood there. The resident responded that he wanted to see what his mentor saw. "I'm not looking. I'm listening," Scalea said.

As a patient or family member, you need your doctor or nurse to be clear and truthful. The message needs to be direct and in everyday speech. In another instance, Dr. Scalea had to tell a mother that her son died. The surgical resident who worked with Scalea in the operating room asked if he could be the one to deliver the bad news. "Sure, I'll just sit to the side," Scalea said. The resident used many words to describe how injured her son had been, how they had tried to save him in the operating room, and then stood up to leave. "Wait," Dr. Scalea said. He walked over, sat down, and held the mother's two hands. "Do you realize that your son has died?" She had not. It is critical for doctors and nurses to be clear.

This is a common problem. A hospital worker frequently involved with death and dying did not initially get clear answers when her husband was hospitalized. "When my husband Sam was on a respirator after a 20-minute resuscitation, I was bombarded with technical talk about EEG activity and brain function. I was confused. Was he 'dead' or wasn't he? After a day of this, a neurologist sat down with me in a private room and said, 'Sam left us yesterday. What we have now is not Sam but a shell. There is no brain activity. You'll need to make a decision about when you want to take him off the respirator.' He sat patiently and allowed me to ask as many questions as I needed. I was very grateful to have it explained to me so clearly and succinctly, yet so thoughtfully and with obvious consideration for my feelings. I didn't need to agonize any more about what I knew had to be done."

Based on my experience in a medical oncology practice, I have some thoughts about humanism and healing. When I had bad news to deliver, it was best to hold the patient's hand. Touch has power. When giving bad news, it is important to be clear. The patient has already guessed his situation, so the doctor should not try to avoid the truth. Then, the doctor should immediately explain what is proposed as next steps. This is absolutely essential. This part must not wait for another day. The patient needs to hear it right now to focus on the hope of a new treatment or plan, even if that means hospice.

On a related note, this apocryphal story is said to have occurred at a famous hospital. A world-renowned cardiac surgeon and his retinue of young doctors-in-training flocked into a patient's room. Standing at the foot of the bed with the others standing silently behind and around him, all in their white coats, the surgeon explained to the man lying in the bed that he needed a heart valve replacement. He told the man about the risks of not proceeding promptly with the surgery and also the risks of the surgery and its aftermath. The surgeon announced that he would perform the surgery first thing tomorrow morning. The patient thanked him but said he needed to talk to his doctor before agreeing to the surgery. The expert was clearly annoyed that his expertise was being questioned. "What is your doctor's name?" "Dr. Hamilton." "Tell me his phone number and I will call him." "I don't know." "Well how can I call him?" the surgeon growled. "Well, he's here in the room – right over there." "He" was the third-year medical student, the only one on the team who had taken the time to have a serious in-depth conversation with the patient. He was the only one who listened to the patient as a person with all of his desires for life and his concerns for family and others. The patient only had a sense of rapport with the student. The surgeon and his retinue left, and the student remained behind. After the student and patient talked, the surgery was soon scheduled for the next day.

A good physician knows that medicine is a "calling." This doctor understands that he or she wields great power through his or her knowledge but is always humble. He probably knows, at least intuitively, what Ambroise Paré, a French surgeon of the early 1500s, wrote: *"Je le pansai, Dieu le guérit"* ("I bandaged him, God healed him."[24]) I suspect this is the view of many physicians; that they can only do so much, and the rest is up to the patient's body and a higher power.

The art of medicine – the art required to become a healer – is not necessarily innate. It takes learning and experience. Not so much book learning but observation of positive role models. When those role models abound, the healing art is much easier to develop and put into practice.

A good physician also takes to heart the saying in Luke 12:48: "Much will be required from everyone to whom much has been given. But even more will be demanded from the one to whom much has been entrusted."

When I became a second-year resident at Yale New Haven Hospital, I asked Jerome Beloff, MD, the professor in charge of the emergency department, how, as a pediatrician previously in private practice for many years, he could listen well to his patient or the parent when there were so many disruptions and time constraints. He offered advice that I tried to follow thereafter throughout my career. When he closed the door to the examining room, he made a conscious commitment to shut off everything other than his patient. This meant no interruptions for a certain amount of time. The patient (and often the parent) should know that he was completely theirs. It was their time. He sat down, listened, and made close eye contact with the child and with the parent. He made every effort to not dwell on other problems or issues that he encountered earlier in the day at work or at home. And if he unexpectedly stumbled onto to a new but non-urgent problem with the patient but did not have enough time to spend that day, he simply told the patient to come back again in a day or two to explore it together in-depth. This was much better, he said, then trying to deal with it in a rush. I found that his advice worked well, but in truth, there were certainly times when it was hard to stay focused on the patient rather than some other event from earlier in the day or still to happen after the patient's visit.

Dr. Rachel Naomi Remen, in her book *My Grandfather's Blessings,* wrote, "As a young doctor, I thought that serving life was a thing of drama and action and split-second judgment calls. A question of going sleepless and riding in ambulances and outwitting the angel of death. A role open only to those who have prepared themselves for years. Service was larger than ordinary life, and those who served were larger than life also. But I know now that this is only the least part of the nature of service. That service is small and quiet and everywhere. That far more often we serve by who we are and not what we know... Many simple, ordinary things that we do can affect those around us in profound ways: the unexpected phone call, the brief touch, the willingness to listen generously, the warm smile or wink of recognition...." [25]

When I was admitted to medical school, a close friend of my parents gave me a reproduction of a deeply moving painting called *The Doctor,* which was painted in 1887 by Sir Luke Fildes and is currently hanging in the Tate Museum in London.[26] (Image ©Tate with permission of The Tate Gallery.)

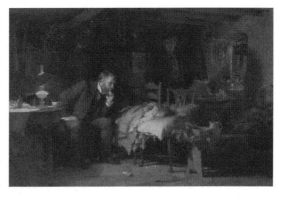

The painting shows a child lying on two chairs in a humble home. The doctor sits nearby looking at her intently. On an adjacent table are a mortar and pestle, presumably used to create a medication. The mother sits at a table behind the child, her head down in her hands, probably sobbing. The father stands beside her with his hand on her shoulder, offering her comfort. The power of the painting is the gaze of the doctor on his patient. Now is the place, the time, the person – he has no other thoughts or concerns except to assist her back to health if he possibly can. We do not know the medical problem, but we can infer that it is serious. And we do not know the outcome, although there may be a clue because through the window comes a faint ray of light.

I did not fully appreciate the implications of this work of art when I first received it, but I came to understand that this physician was a healer.

He had listened; he was nonjudgmental; he had earned trust. He has done his best but, like Paré, understood that he alone would not be her cause of cure, should a cure ensue. He understands that he is but a humble person entrusted with the most important of all missions – to assist others to find health. He has done his best, and in doing so, exemplifies the characteristics of a healer.

The general practitioners of my grandfather's period had few medications to give, few tests to run and limited surgical technologies, but like the doctor in the painting by Sir Luke Fields, they had compassion, patience and empathy. My grandfather listened deeply in a nonjudgmental fashion. He was well loved by his patients even though he often could not cure their diseases or injuries. But he was still a healer.

Medicine changed as it became tethered to economic considerations. Today, those powerful financial forces have resulted in little time for listening. Instead, medicine today focuses on the technical, the tests, the images and the procedures. Certainly these are and can be useful, but it has come at the loss of the healer – a loss of great import.

Dr. Jeff Kane describes this change well: "I've been dismayed to see its aura fade as health care devolved from the humane service to a cooler commercial enterprise. Remnants of its original juice will always persist though and will be the source of genuine reform.... It's the alleviation of suffering through personal contact alone. Applied skillfully it can transform the medical examining room from the utilitarian cubicle it's become back into the intimate sanctuary it once was, a healing temple arguably more potent than drugs or surgery."[18]

The good primary care physician is one well-versed in the science of medicine, is up-to-date on the new evidence-based approaches to care delivery, listens deeply, uses an integrative approach and has the knowledge, experience and desire to be a healer. I would add that being a doctor is a privilege. Doctors are given that privilege as a result of medical school and residency training, years of experience and a willingness to put patient care above all else. It is a special – indeed, sacred – privilege. Physicians need to always remember that it is a privilege granted by the patient, each and every time they have an encounter. It is a privilege that the patient can choose to retract.

You, as a patient, should always feel it is your absolute right to retract that privilege and move on to another physician who offers you the medical skills, plus the healing care, that you deserve and have every right to expect.

You need and deserve a superb clinician who is also a healer. You can — with the comments above in mind — observe your primary care physician in action when you arrive with a problem. Does he or she listen attentively? Allow you to fully explain the situation? Treat you as a unique individual? Offer a suggested course of action only after understanding your unique needs and concerns? Quickly give you the sense of trust and commitment you need and deserve? If you do not feel satisfied as you reviewed these characteristics, the PCP is probably not for you and will not be the best fit if you develop a more serious problem.

PART II

FACTS, FRUSTRATIONS, CONSUMERISM
AND GOVERNMENT INCURSIONS

Part II explores several attempts to improve healthcare through the medical home concept and introduces readers to population health as an alternative to individual episodic care. We will discuss the conflict between physician and nurse practitioner organizations and how that impacts patients and overall healthcare. Part II wraps up with a discussion of how the intense primary care physician frustrations have impacted the rest of us while patients are no longer willing to be "patient."

Chapter Six

PRIMARY CARE: JUST THE FACTS (AND FIGURES)

Some thoughts from Dr. Andy Lazris, a geriatrician and primary care physician in practice for twenty five years. "We are getting pummeled; time is being taken from us while our tasks, especially non-clinical and regulatory ones, are increasing. That leaves us little time to sit down casually with our patients and really talk about what's going on. The end result is mutual dis-satisfaction, worse care, and higher cost due to testing, referrals, and hospitalization. In residency, one of my wise mentors taught me a lesson I have been using for 25 years: the best visit is to look your patient in the eye and let them do the talking. It's their visit, and it's their agenda, and the more you talk the least satisfied they will be. That ability is being stripped away. When I started practice one doctor said to me that the best visit is to order a bunch of tests, prescriptions and referrals and then your patient thinks you are really helping them. But today's patient is much wiser; they don't like that approach. They like a doctor who can listen and who responds to their agenda. Sadly, in today's world, most practices are gravitating to the short visit/high intervention strategy that has become the norm."[27]

The Shortage of Primary Care Physicians

Why it is that America has only 30 percent primary care physicians? There are many reasons, but it is fundamentally tied to the insurance system that rewards specialty practice and those who do procedures more than those who do more cognitively-based work. Reimbursements for PCPs have remained stable for some years, so for the PCP to cover rising overhead costs and still continue to earn about $150,000 to $180,000 per year (compared to twice that for specialists), he or she needs to see many patients per day. That leads to the poor quality care described previously.

I do not want to advocate for a particular income for primary care physicians or any other physician. The average income for a PCP today is certainly enough keep the wolf from the door. But I will remind you that a PCP does not get started on a career until about age 30 and does so after many years of schooling and training, which adds up to an educational debt load of nearly $200,000. On top of that, the hours are long. Most PCPs spend 60-70 hours per week in the office and then have night call. More importantly, they have a high responsibility: your health. I would imagine that, like most of us, the PCP would like to earn much more than they do, but money was not the driver of why they entered medicine in the first place. They want to maintain the income they have now, but that means seeing more patients per day.

Frustrated that they are on a treadmill and not practicing the level of care that they would like to offer, many PCPs are leaving their long-time typical private practice and joining the local hospital as a salaried employee. Others are simply retiring early. Just a few years ago, about two-thirds of PCPs were in private practice, but today that has been reduced to about one-third and continues to fall. Practices that were always physician-owned are rapidly dwindling. Why this switch? Some say it is financial pressure, frustration with insurers' requirements for getting preauthorization for various tests and procedures, lifestyle desires, and an increasing desire among newer graduates to avoid administrative responsibilities.

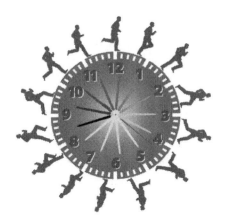

But employment rather than private practice has its disadvantages as well. The top four complaints among employed physicians, according to a Medscape survey, were "being bossed by a less educated administrator," not being able to make decisions about staff, having limited authority over billing, and being essentially "forced" to order tests using new hospital-based equipment or technology. Multiple hospital-employed physicians have told me about expectations placed on them to hit a target per quarter for MRIs, CT and PET scans – an expectation that can at best be described as unethical.

Medical students are cognizant of the issues and see that primary care physicians appear to be on a never-ending production line with less income, more responsibilities, longer hours and substantial night call duties, yet are frustrated that they cannot give the best possible care to their patients. Add the fact that almost all graduating students today have substantial debt, and it is not surprising they gravitate toward specialty care. Many who do enter primary care are international medical graduates who do their post graduate clinical training in the United States. During my interviews, PCPs generally agreed that the trend toward choosing specialty care was not because of debt nor expected income but rather not wanting the frustration and the "treadmill" that seems to be part of today's PCP practice.

All of this has resulted in major declines in medical students entering primary care. Recall the estimate that by 2025 there will be a PCP shortage of 52,000 doctors. The number assumes PCPs will continue to have 2,500 patients in their practice – a number that is too high for the best quality of care. Bring that number down and the shortage number goes up substantially.

An Average Day for a PCP

Not surprisingly, the PCPs I interviewed differed in their descriptions of an "average day," but not that much. A good example: "I can divide my patient visits into three groups. A third have acute simple stuff like strep throat or an abscess. A third have well-controlled chronic issues like diabetes or hypertension or are well and coming in for an annual exam. The final third have complex chronic illnesses like poorly-controlled hypertension or out-of-control diabetes." Most said they can take care of "simple stuff" over the phone without the need for a visit, but others said they ask the patients to come in since they do not get paid for phone consults.

Most said stress was a factor in at about 20-30 percent of visits. Others gave a number closer to 50 percent. One suggested: "If I probed further, I bet stress or anxiety is a contributing factor in many more." About 50 percent of patients with chronic illnesses have a stress or anxiety-inducing component that exacerbates an otherwise stable status. Another noted that many acute problems are an overlay on a chronic issue, and stress is often a major inciting factor.

Dr. R. J. Baron published an article on how a primary care physician spends his or her time. He is part of a Philadelphia area internal medicine group practice with an active caseload of 8,840 patients divided across the equivalent of four full-time physicians each working 50-60 hours per week. The office has 3.5 full-time support staff per physician. Each physician handles 24 telephone calls and 17 emails, reviews 20 laboratory tests reports, 11 imaging reports and 14 consultation notes and processes 12 prescription refills each day in addition to seeing patients. It is clear from this report that the PCPs spend a lot of time in clinically-relevant work not directly associated with a patient visit, which is the only activity that generates an insurance reimbursement. Not noted was the substantial time spent in non-clinical requirements, such as completing insurance forms.[28]

An Average Day For a PCP --- Other Than Seeing Patients

Clinically Relevant Work
- 24 Telephone calls
- 17 Emails
- 20 Laboratory reports
- 11 Imaging reports
- 14 Consultation notes
- 12 Prescription refills (in addition to those written during a patient visit)

Non Clinically Relevant
- Insurer requirements
- Electronic Medical Record issues

Needless to say, it is difficult to provide your best primary care when you are spending your day doing everything but that.

The Patient – PCP Ratio

How many patients can a PCP reasonably see? In my in-depth interviews, PCPs gave widely divergent responses ranging from 500 to 3,000 – or more. Yet many were clearly conflicted. Some said they can manage about 2,000 with little difficulty, but then they observed elsewhere in the conversation that they have no time for communicating with the specialist or hospitalist. A general consensus appears to be that 1,500 patients is the upper limit, provided it is a practice in which the PCP has gotten to know most of the patients over many years. Otherwise, a lower number seems appropriate. For example, one highly-experienced PCP noted he has about 1,500 patients, including a few sick patients he must see frequently and others he only sees every few years when issues arise. But even at 1,500, he still spends the full day seeing patients with added time each evening completing his electronic medical records.

Beyond that, the PCPs say 1,000 would mean much better care, but is not possible. They need to have about 2,500 patients and 25 visits per day to cover overhead and maintain an income of about $150,000 to $180,000. All want to keep some time each day for same-day appointments and minor emergencies, plus time slots for patients seen today who need to return in a few days for a follow-up. The pressure to see 25 patients per day means it is difficult to hold a few slots each day for urgent problems. The patients are still seen but are "squeezed in," which happens to the detriment of the doctor, the patient with an urgent issue, and the patients scheduled immediately before and after the urgent patient.

All of the PCPs agreed that if the population is largely geriatric – meaning more likely to have multiple chronic conditions – then a lower maximum is necessary. One primary care group (discussed in detail in a later chapter) limits their practice to geriatric patients in a Medicare Advantage program and holds the number of patients per physician to about 400. At this number, they can give good care, have high patient satisfaction, and keep the *total* cost of care well below the local and national averages for older patients.

Given these examples, it appears that, in a practice comprised of a wide range of patient ages and problems, there should be about 1,000 or fewer patients. For a practice with many healthy younger patients or one organized like a medical home with a team approach, 1,500 might be acceptable. For a geriatric-oriented practice, 400-500 should be the maximum.

To continue the discussion on LinkedIn, I asked, "How many patients can a PCP safely care for each day?" There were more than 50 responses. Of course, the answer is, "It depends." It depends on the mix of patients and their needs. But the respondents focused on *time* and the importance of time to fully and compassionately treat each patient properly. The patient needs "faith in the doctor, which when present, slashes the illness in half," one doctor said. Developing faith takes time. Another PCP stated that "patients are not products on an assembly line that must fit into specified compartments as the business model dictates. Time is what affords the physician the ability to utilize all of his or her experience and medical expertise in the most efficient manner to benefit the patient." Another urged fellow PCPs to learn how to lead and function in a team-based setting, thereby empowering each team member to rise to the peak of individual expertise while allowing the PCP to devote more time to the complex. Consistent with the team concept, another stated that PCPs today spend only 20-30 percent of their time in face-to-face contact with their patients. He urged PCPs to delegate the data entry responsibilities that today consume 40-50 percent of a PCP's time. But as another noted, PCPs (and physicians in general) have not been educated and trained in the team-based care approach nor in team leadership – an experience and skill critical to engaging a team in the office.

A general theme in the discussion was that PCPs need to overcome their reluctance to enter the political arena. They need to stop blaming others for the lack of time with their patients and instead join their state medical societies, specialty organizations such as the American College of Physicians and the American Medical Association, and through them, lobby aggressively for the time needed to care for their patients.

An article in the *Annals of Family Medicine* by Dr. J. Altshuler and others[29] sought to estimate a reasonably-sized patient panel for a PCP with team-based task delegation similar to the patient-centered medical home model. Using published estimates of the time needed by a PCP to provide preventive, chronic and acute care, they modeled how panel sizes would change if a portion of the work in each of the three categories was delegated to team members. If there was no delegation of work, as has been typical in PCP practices for decades, the data suggest that a patient panel size of about 983 is the maximum, not too far from my own estimate of 1,000 based on the various interviews. With varying levels of delegation, their model panels ranged from 1,387 to 1,947 patients. This analysis suggests that a primary care physician can care for more than 1,000 patients with a well-oiled team-based medical home practice. It does not address the question of whether the team can practice true "population health," meaning the PCP and team reach out proactively to all members of the patient panel to address high quality preventive care rather than wait for the patient to arrive at the office with a problem.

Colleague to Colleague Advice and Interaction

With a reasonably-sized practice, the PCP can have more time. As stated before, this is important time needed to listen, think, prevent and coordinate. And it allows for collegial interaction – a quick discussion or a more formalized interaction. PCPs in solo or group practice today usually do not have the time to interact with each other when they encounter an unusual or challenging situation. During medical school and training at a teaching hospital, there are always others around to interact with, which is an important part of the educational process, but it is often lost once doctors are out in the community. Those who practice within an academic medical center make use of this opportunity regularly, perhaps while in the cafeteria or pre/post a conference. Called a "curbside consult," it means taking a few minutes to bounce an idea or issue off a colleague. It can be highly valuable and lead to better care. But in a fast-paced private practice in the community environment, this is generally not possible.

"As long as patients visit their primary care clinicians for front-line help with undifferentiated symptoms, disabling chronic conditions, and for end-of-life decision-making, uncertainty will remain an insistent companion," says Lucia Sommers in a book about how she and her colleagues explored collaborative engagement with case-based uncertainty in the setting of small groups of clinicians. They suggest that although time to listen and think is critical, the "thinking" part needs both time and a *different type* of thinking – an opportunity for augmenting the traditional model of the individual physician thinking alone with a collegial one where physicians reflect and learn together, particularly when tackling case-based uncertainty. Briefly, they organized the routine gathering of small groups of PCPs to discuss challenging cases. Part of the process was to increase comfort levels in being able to say to a colleague, "I'm stumped; let me tell you about my conundrum." Their observations suggest that this approach opens the mind to new considerations of diagnosis and treatment, improves decision making and reduces uncertainty.[30] But of course, this collaborative discussion takes time. It gives one more reason why it is imperative that the PCP (or any physician) has enough time to give the highest quality of care, yet not enough time to be wasteful of resources.

PCPs with a challenging case often would like the opportunity to test a hypothesis, diagnosis or treatment plan with a colleague, but time and distance limit their ability to do so. However, brief, pointed interaction is a commonplace approach when colleagues are readily available – in the hospital cafeteria, coffee shop or hallway. In an effort to make this "curbside consult" concept available to any practicing PCP, RubiconMD connects a PCP with a specialist who responds to a brief query about a patient with a brief written response – all done by computer and over the Internet. The query does not include patient-specific identifying characteristics. Rather, it offers only relevant history, examination, laboratory or imaging data. The specialist responds with a few paragraphs in a way that might prompt further testing or questioning of the patient, or it might recommend that the patient needs a specialist referral.

This business model began with the observations that 40 percent of referrals from PCPs to specialists are poorly timed or not needed, 40 percent of referrals never happen, and 20 percent of referrals result in duplicate or unnecessary imaging or tests. RubiconMD hopes to convince insurers or businesses/corporations to pay for the specialist commentary to reduce the number of referrals (and hence total costs), limit the amount of testing (again, costs), direct referrals to the most appropriate type of specialist, and send referrals with the relevant tests, images, and lab data.

My conclusion from the data I reviewed and my in-depth interviews is that the number of patients most primary care physicians have today – 2,500 or more – is far too many for one PCP to manage adequately. At that number, they tend to refer many patients to specialists in order to manage their patient load. If the PCP had more time with each patient, those referrals would be unnecessary in many, if not most, cases. A maximum size patient panel should be about 1,000, but even 1,000 is too many if the panel has many individuals with complex chronic illnesses, which are generally older patients who also may have hearing, vision or cognitive issues as well. Of course, reducing the number of patients per doctor means either lower income (not very satisfying for the doctor) or a revision of the payment system (not likely from Medicare or most commercial insurers.) I will review a number of approaches as we continue and I will offer some personal recommendations.

CHAPTER SEVEN

TEAMS ARE IMPORTANT FOR HEALTHCARE: NURSE PRACTITIONERS, PHYSICIAN ASSISTANTS AND PRIMARY CARE PHYSICIANS

Can the use of nurse practitioners (NP) or physician assistants (PA) help address the PCP shortage? This is an issue that, unfortunately, is fraught with contentious debate by some who are concerned about losing their "turf," combined with a general lack of understanding about what superior primary care is and how it can benefit health, wellness and illness.

Can They Replace the PCP? Augment the PCP?

The PCPs I interviewed had various opinions. All appreciated the training and skills of nurse practitioners and physician assistants. Many worked with NPs or PAs as part of their team. One group has an NP assigned to a local nursing home and finds the patient care is much better as a result. The same group has a hospital inpatient NP who works to ensure good discharge instructions and follow-up and is well-versed in the community services that patients may need after discharge. Another is in a group of two physicians and three nurse practitioners, each with their own patients but interacting daily as a team. But none of the PCPs thought NPs should have the same scope of practice rights as physicians. They emphasized that too many physicians have demeaned NPs and PAs and that this was inappropriate. But many felt the amount of training for NPs or PAs was not adequate to replace the PCP, leaving them inexperienced and not able to function independently. One PCP observed that the NPs he knew tended to either minimize or maximize findings, and sometimes serious problems were left undiagnosed or simple illnesses were over tested. He said, "It's like medical internship – you don't know what you don't know and hence need supervision." In general, PCPs found NPs and PAs to be great for acute, straightforward illnesses, ongoing management of chronic diseases, patient follow-up and nutrition and medication compliance. But most PCPs would not use them to do key diagnostics of complex chronic illnesses.

During the interviews, younger physicians tended to accept a wider role for both NPs and PAs. They noted that PCPs have resisted the NP scope-of-practice issue, but given that there are not enough PCPs, they believe there is a need to use everyone effectively. They agree that NP training is not adequate for full scope of practice, but they support more on-the-job training for NPs and PAs rather than trying to "shut them down" outright. In fact, they observed that NPs have an ability to connect and listen to patients. One PCP thought this is because they were nurses by original training and have learned empathy.

A recent national survey of both physicians and nurse practitioners published in *The New England Journal of Medicine* revealed the wide divergence of views on this issue. More than 90 percent of NPs worked in a setting with a physician, whereas 41 percent of doctors worked with an NP. Also, NPs were more likely to respond that NPs could lead a medical home, should be allowed to have hospital-admitting privileges and should be paid the same for equivalent work. Two-thirds of physicians agreed with a statement that doctors provide higher quality examinations than NPs, and only one quarter of NPs agreed with that statement. It was clear from the survey that physicians and NPs do not agree about what the roles of each should be in the future provider workforce.[31]

A physician in a group of doctors and nurse practitioners told me "We all work as a team. One problem a lot of docs have with NP's is that of pay equity. In fact, our NP's make similar money to some community primary care docs, which is hardly fair given the amount of training docs have to endure. That's an issue that will eventually have to be resolved if NP's and docs are going to work in harmony, as well they should."

From one patient's perspective: "I have to wonder about breaking through cultural norms. I think that many people believe only the doctor can give the best advice, and they will think that having a PA, NP or other health care professional consultation means they aren't getting the best care. I think it will be up to the PCP to convince his patients that the health care professionals on his 'team' have been selected to optimize actual health care delivery and not just 'sick care.' In April 2011, after my father's six-month illness and near-death situations, working on major project at work, and a close friend's death, I saw the PA in my PCP's office for a physical because the PCP was too busy to see me for a month or two. I wasn't thrilled but complied. She asked how I was doing. Unexpectedly, I started crying and pouring out my story of my father's illness, stress at work and the death of my beloved friend. She didn't try to stop or interrupt and listened until I stopped talking and asked how she could help. We talked a few minutes about what to do, and she offered a follow-up appointment. I felt better after my 'purge' and her validation that I really had been through a difficult and stressful time. I had been reluctant to see the PA instead of the PCP but not again. I don't think I would have gotten the same amount of time and attention from him. *It simply wasn't his to give.* So educating the patients on how a team can work together for better health care will be important, and I'm not sure who can successfully accomplish it other than the PCP."

At AbsoluteCARE (see Chapter 13 for more details), the provider team is a physician or an NP, plus a case manager, nurse and medical assistant, all working as a team. Two teams share a work area – one team with a PCP lead, the other with an NP. The PCP is readily available to the NP as needed. Dr. Gregory Foti, the physician medical director, told me, "I want to empower the NPs here. We work as a team. I will give her extra support with issues that she feels challenged with. I want her to know that I am here for her – for any questions or support that she needs. We each have our skills and attributes; she is great at building trust and relationships. Our system is that I am the director but it is not hierarchical; we are all in this together to give outstanding care."

Dr. Andrew Morris-Singer, founder and president of Primary Care Progress (see Chapter 16), says their organization is completely inclusive. About 50 percent of their chapters across the country include NPs and PAs. "We can understand, respect and leverage each other's talents," he says. "The key is teams, not separatism." He is in favor of advancing scope-of-practice laws for NPs but for the purpose of working in a team, not independently.

"We don't need more 'Lone Rangers' [or ones who work alone rather than as a well-oiled team], whether that be NPs or MDs. Unfortunately, there are many extremist positions with the leaders on both sides taking pot shots at each other. This is not valuable. They don't seem to realize that there is a huge group of physicians, NPs and PAs who like to work together."

Rebecca Sedillo, FNP is a recent graduate and now working in a rural healthcare center. She wrote, "My involvement with Primary Care Progress and the community of primary care faculty and students at the University of California San Francisco has been healing. Instead of being greeted with skepticism and lack of awareness about my role as a nurse practitioner, I have been invited by my primary care colleagues to join a movement and be part of a community. My confidence grew as I started to believe that just as primary care providers deserve respect and recognition for their important contributions to healthcare today, nurse practitioners belong in the primary care movement, too. We have plenty of work ahead of us to strengthen relationships between the nursing and medical field, across healthcare professions, and between primary care and other specialties. But in the meantime, supportive communities, such as the one we are building through Primary Care Progress, will keep us committed, inspired, and compelled to do what we are meant to do."[32]

Unfortunately, some physicians and NPs take extreme positions. In my view, it is better to work together, find the middle ground and maximize the value and work of each. It is also important to recognize that medical care delivery is changing. In the future, the PCP working alone will transform into the PCP working as part of a team, which might include an NP, PA, nurse, case manager and medical assistant. Each can – and should – do what they do best. When that happens, patient care improves substantially and becomes true health care rather than just medical care.

CHAPTER EIGHT

THE FUTURE IS NOW: ACCOUNTABLE CARE ORGANIZATIONS, THE MEDICAL HOME AND POPULATION HEALTH

I will venture a guess that 99 percent of you reading this get your medical care in an episodic fashion, which means you interact with the medical care system only when you have a problem. For some of you, but probably not the majority, you visit your PCP for an "annual checkup." At this session, your doctor may spend some time discussing preventive care with behavior modification for weight or smoking and medications to counteract screening abnormalities such as high blood pressure or high cholesterol. Your PCP may also administer immunizations at this time and encourage you to get a mammogram or colonoscopy. You may find the visit pleasant, especially if nothing adverse is discovered. During the appointment, you interact briefly with the front office clerk who registered you, the nurse who took your blood pressure and weight, the doctor, and then the billing clerk on the way out. But most likely, all of the medical part of the visit was with the doctor and did not include follow-up from anyone else. In short, it was not a true team but rather a group of individuals with a specific role to aid the doctor in the process of giving you care. Further, despite the fact that you might have various health risk factors or even a simmering chronic illness, there was no proactive approach on the part of the doctor's office during the course of the prior year. The doctor and assistants only moved into action after you arrived for your annual visit.

Patient-centered medical home

The "patient-centered medical home," or PCMH, offers the possibility of better care and is essentially what I have advocated throughout this book. The concept is to provide comprehensive care to patients by offering proactive and ongoing care management rather than the typical reactive care practiced by most PCPs today. This includes compliance with preventive screenings, rapid access for acute problems, and evidence-based management of chronic illnesses with care coordination. Among other aspects, the PCMH concept emphasizes the team approach and transfers some authority and responsibility to other team members, thereby reducing the workload of the PCP and improving the quality of care. For example, the team keeps records – preferably electronically – that indicate a patient arriving for a visit for one reason should be reminded by the medical assistant to schedule a colonoscopy. With this record in hand, the receptionist taking the appointment phone call can sometimes do this over the phone and offer to set up the appointment for the patient at that moment. This type of proactive approach greatly improves compliance with basic preventive measures and ensures that tests to monitor ongoing issues are completed and ready for review when the patient sees the doctor. Under this model, the PCP is still the captain of the ship, but the team now functions like a real team. The National Committee for Quality Assurance (NCQA) offers guidance to PCPs who wish to have their practice certified.[33]

Consider this physician's transition: Peter Anderson, MD, would have quit medicine in 2002 if he had not had an alternative. Run ragged by his role as a primary care physician who served as a "gatekeeper" to his patients, frustrated by having invested early in electronic medical records yet working longer and harder, and getting poorer as he added staffing to comply with administrative responsibilities foisted upon him by payers, he was depressed and looking for an exit strategy. Instead of practicing efficient and effective healthcare, Anderson says his goal became "seeing as many patients as I could without making a mistake." His office was in chaos, two of his nurses were openly threatening to quit, and his patients were dissatisfied. Besides that, he did not know them. "I had to focus more attention on the EMR [electronic medical record] than on the patient and lost patient interaction," he says. "That loss of connection was disheartening, but you lived and died by that EMR chart.[34]"

He realized that to give the attention his patients needed, he should give more "face time," but he could not afford the additional time and still cover his overhead costs. At some point, he had that "eureka moment" when he began to realize that what he really needed to do was not try to run harder (or exit primary care altogether) but work more efficiently using the members of his office staff.

He began to have his nurses interview patients upon arrival. When he entered the exam room, the nurse would explain to Anderson in front of the patient what she had just learned. Anderson would then ask additional questions, do an appropriate exam and develop a plan. As this happened, the nurse typed details into the EMR. He would briefly tell the patient the plan and then leave the room. The nurse would go over the details of the plan in much greater detail with the patient, ensuring that it was fully understood and asking if the patient had additional questions. Meanwhile, Dr. Anderson moved to the next exam room, where another nurse and patient were ready. At the end of the day, he reviewed each patient's EMR for accuracy and completeness.

With this new approach, he could see more patients per day and increase revenue yet spend fewer hours in the office. Most importantly, even though his time in the exam room was shorter, he spent more time interacting with patients and less time with paperwork.

In an effort to get back to what made medicine attractive to him initially – consulting, cajoling, and helping his patients – he had to delegate, which is one of the main tenets of the patient-centered medical home concept.

According to the principles laid out by primary care professional societies, patient-centered medical homes should have these characteristics: a personal physician, physician-directed medical practice, whole-person orientation, coordinated care, quality and safety, enhanced access and adequate payment.

A summary of the jointly-developed principles of the medical home model of the American Academy of Family Practice, The American College of Medicine and the American Osteopathic Association, in part, reads: "At its core is an ongoing partnership between each person and a specially trained primary care physician. This new model provides modern conveniences, like email communication and same-day appointments; quality ratings and pricing information; and secure online tools to help consumers manage their health information, review the latest medical findings and make informed decisions. Consumers receive reminders about necessary appointments and screenings, as well as other support to help them and their families manage chronic conditions such as diabetes or heart disease. ... the primary care physician makes sure the [team is] working together to meet all of the patient's needs in an integrated, 'whole person' fashion."[35]

But this is an impossible set of criteria to meet fully unless the payment model changes. Most physicians could not begin to meet these criteria and still stay in practice. Certainly, a change in the style of practice, which uses team members to the full extent of their training and education, will not only make the physician's time less hectic but also improve quality of care and reduce costs. However, the team members need to be paid. More work, even if accomplished by team members with lower salaries, still must be reimbursed.

In this model, the team members are expected to serve at the top of their professional expertise, thus reducing some of the work of the PCP. Some doctors recommend that medical assistants, rather than nurses, take the patient's history and present it to the physician at exam time. This is fine for collecting routine information but not for diagnosis. It is just as inappropriate to employ someone without detailed medical training to take the history as it is to ask patients to wait in the exam room in a gown before the doctor has met with them to take the history. This idea may speed up the process but is incredibly disrespectful of the patient. I imagine Dr. Anderson's approach is more efficient. It makes better use of the skills and compassion of nurses and is effective from a biomedical approach to care. However, I wonder if it allows the doctor to take the time to interact with the patient – to listen deeply and find the hidden meaning of the medical symptom. Perhaps the nurse does this, which is fine. But to me, it removes the most critical and enjoyable element of being a physician: the relationship between doctor and patient. He would counter that he actually has more time which is meaningful time now than before.

The PCMH may not be appropriate in all circumstances. Largely, it has been tested in settings of highly-integrated care systems with a single payer. Considering that only a small percentage of patients consume the vast majority of health care dollars, this type of system would be most valuable for them. The PCMH is likely of less importance for many others, although it might be important to ensure better preventive medicine. A recent study published in the *Journal of the American Medical Association* compared 32 small and medium-sized community practices that followed the PCMH concept to 29 that did not. Combined, they served about 110,000 patients and multiple participating health plans. The PCMH practices all achieved the NCQA certification, but after three years, there were not any reductions in hospital admissions, ER visits or total costs to the system. Of eleven quality measures, only one showed a substantial improvement compared to the other practices.[36] This raises the questions of when and how the PCMH concept can be best utilized.[37]

From my PCP interviews, it was clear that some were enthusiastic and others simply did not know what a medical home model was. One PCP said, "Our practice is working toward it. To us, it is just about good care. It is what we should do anyway. If you're doing good medicine, it is a medical home. But to be certified, we need to keep good records. Some of the NCQA requirements are extra work or are basically 'process' measures rather than 'outcome' measures and may not be that critical." Another doctor, who is part of a group of PCPs, suggested, "I am not convinced that checking boxes on 150 elements makes a practice better, but I do certainly believe that many of the elements of PCMH are fundamental to excellence – continuity, access, coordination of care, identification of high risk and management accordingly. The NCQA has made PCMH a business and convinced everyone that accreditation is of paramount importance. I'm not so sure. We're working our way there to make sure we don't miss a big financial opportunity, but there are a number of checkboxes that are just not necessary."

Another PCP said "We belong to an ACO and medical home, and neither has been very useful to us or our patients; in fact, often they add to our work burden and they stress out our patients. Maybe one day they will be better, but often less trained people going into the homes of older patients are quicker to panic (their pressure is too high, sugars too high, too short of breath) about issues that are fairly stable, and people go to the hospital with more rapidity than if they were seeing us or not being so closely monitored. I believe that over-monitoring the elderly can be dangerous, and sometimes that is what happens."

Some said they thought they were essentially practicing as a medical home, that it was a good model, and that they hoped to achieve certification.

Others said that given the time constraints, it was impossible to do more than they did now. Those who were using the concept or getting started talked about changing how they use nurses in the practice, such as tracking patients' medications, visits and immunization records. They now have regular team meetings to review how new roles are working. Some have extended hours into the evenings or weekends, and some do a limited amount of home visits. Overall, the responses were generally positive for those invested in the concept and quizzical for those who were not involved. A clinic for those with multiple chronic illnesses (AbsoluteCARE) uses the concept effectively and will be discussed in Chapter 13.

As one PCP blogged: "The impending shortage of PCPs constitutes a national emergency. In order to provide the growing Medicare population with compassionate, effective healthcare at a sustainable cost, seniors will need stable relationships with PCPs who can function as their strategic medical consultants, collaborate in helping to meet healthcare goals, and provide emotional support.

For instance, consider the kinds of issues I routinely address as a general internist for older adults: Following up on 6+ chronic conditions and 12+ medications in an integrated whole-person fashion. Following-up on the work of multiple specialists, many of whom hadn't explained their thinking to the patient and family. Yes, these specialists should get better at explaining their thinking. No, they will probably not resolve the conflicts between their recommendations and some other specialist's recommendations. Resolving the conflicts is inherent in attempting to follow clinical practice guidelines in patients with multiple conditions. Elderly patients routinely generate a gazillion conflicting clinical practice guidelines. Helping patients and families evaluate the likely benefits and burdens of possible medical approaches. Should that lung nodule be biopsied? Should knee replacement surgery be considered now, or still deferred? So many of the decisions we face have no clear right answer.

Doing this type of PCP work can be extremely rewarding, but it's also cognitively and emotionally demanding."[38]

From this basic thesis, she suggested that, medical home or not, the work is intense. The PCP can be greatly assisted with the PCMH concept, but there still needs to be a limit to how much work the PCP does.

I would restate this as: the PCP needs a lower number of patients in order to serve each patient appropriately. The elements of the "medical home" model make sense but only will improve care when the doctor has time.

Population Health

Population health is a relatively new term for an old idea. Basically, it means taking responsibility for the total health care of a group of individuals, not just care of episodes of sickness when they occur. The triple aim – improved quality, good health, reasonable cost. Episodic care is the essence of what most physicians do today. A person develops chest pain, goes to the doctor (or the ER), is evaluated and then treated. Population health dictates that all patients under the care of that doctor (or group of doctors) have close proactive attention to their disease prevention, along with health and wellness counseling. Those with chronic illness need a proactive approach to discovering and managing the disease before it results in new symptoms. Done correctly, this leads to better health of the entire population and each individual within it, better disease management and lower costs overall.

A "population" might be everyone in a geographic area, a political subdivision, a medical demographic (for example, those with serious medical problems complicated by socioeconomic deprivation), or all the patients in a single doctor's practice. The population health concept is for the health care provider (such as the PCP, NP, PA, group practice) or some other organization (such as a health plan or local hospital) to accept responsibility for the total health management of a specific population. This is much different in concept than being paid for responding only to episodic events. Payment is for the totality of care and is based on outcomes. For example, how good is the control of diabetes or hypertension among these individuals? How successful is the system at preventing obesity, reducing high cholesterol, slowing the progression of osteoporosis or detecting depressive symptoms early?

In practice, it means a group of PCPs take on shared accountability for a population of people. From an insurer's perspective, the population size needs to be more than 5,000 to make it actuarially viable to measure the triple aim of improved quality, improved health and reduced costs. To the extent it works appropriately, this model should enhance the satisfaction and the income of the PCP. Concurrently, it should result in a better system than at present, win the trust of the patients, and keep patients out of the hospital and away from unnecessary specialist visits.

The PCPs are paid to the extent that they increase quality while reducing costs. To do this, the doctors must identify those within the population who are at great risk or are the heaviest users. Under this concept, about 5 percent of patients consume about 50 percent of the total costs of the group. They are sometimes known as "ambulatory ICU patients," and the greatest resources need to be directed toward them. The current quality measures are nationally-accepted, such as diabetes control (HA1c levels that measure blood sugar over time), high blood pressure control, percent of age and gender-appropriate patients who receive mammography or colonoscopy screenings, percent of patients immunized as appropriate, percent of generic prescriptions filled (rather than brand name) and more. Unfortunately, the average PCP practice does not have the resources needed by this high-risk group, such as nutritionists and social workers, and it is not clear that the payers will expend the dollars to make them available, even though used properly it might well reduce their total costs over time.

Carried out to its fullest extent, the population health approach also includes the social, economic, environmental and other elements that contribute to the health of an individual. Ultimately, it is essential to address social inequities related to nutrition, exercise, safety, education and housing, all of which significantly impact health and wellness. Medical care, as generally construed, has a relatively small influence on ultimate health outcomes when compared with other determinants such as socioeconomic status. Nevertheless, it is imperative to address. American medical care has not been nearly as proactive as it could be and should be.

Some PCPs think of population health only in terms of a payment system that compensates for taking risk for quality, health and cost, however defined. It is an insurance model to address the financial implications for managing health rather than only disease. Alternatively, in our current fee-for-service system, it is possible to achieve the same outcomes with a patient-centric approach that focuses heavily on proactively preventing disease, managing existent disease and rarely referring to a specialist.

Assume that a primary care physician has 2,500 patients in his or her practice. Extrapolating from average data across the country, R. Hodach from the American Medical Group Association calculates that this population of 2,500 people would include the following numbers with chronic diseases.[39] The size of these numbers and their relative ranking may surprise you.

Common Chronic Diseases Among an Average of 2,500 Patients	
Chronic Conditions	2,500 Patients
Hyperlipidemia	511
Hypertension	472
Arthritis	381
Anxiety	289
Asthma	183
Diabetes	145
Osteoporosis	140
Chronic Obstructive Pulmonary Disease (COPD)	131
Coronary Artery Disease	120
Depression	118

Of course, these are averages. A specific doctor's practice population would vary widely based on whether it is rural or urban, the population's socioeconomic status and the population's age. For example, a practice that includes mostly geriatric patients would have more individuals with chronic diseases. The point here is that the PCP's team should proactively determine who these patients are and institute medical management now, rather than wait for the patient to arrive at the office with a problem.

It should be possible to assess the health *risk* of a population as well. That 2,500-person population has chronic illnesses, and it also can be expected – again on average – to have 550 individuals who drink alcohol to excess, 275 who smoke and 850 who are at risk for skin cancer. The task in population health is to detect the risk factors, evaluate them and put effective preventive management plans into place. The next table gives the rank order of risk prevalence for a practice of 2,500 individuals.

Risk Prevalence Across a 2,500 Person Population	
Health Risk Category	**2,500 Patients**
Nutrition	2,400
Weight Management	1,600
- Overweight	-825
- Obese	-624
- Extremely Obese	-150
Physical Inactivity	1,200
Chronic Stress	875
Skin Protection	850
Alcohol Excess	550
Injury Prevention	400
Depression Symptoms	300
Smoking	275
Sexual Behaviors	25

In the table, the most common risk factors are related to nutrition and weight management, exercise and stress. Indeed, 2,400 of the 2,500 have a less than favorable nutritional status, 1,600 are overweight, and nearly one-half get too little exercise. These are people ripe for developing diabetes, high blood pressure and coronary artery disease, with the possibility of heart attacks and strokes. Plus, stress in a quarter of the population exacerbates disease progression. Smoking, although lower on the list, has a high propensity to cause disease and death. The doctor (and the associated team) in this new model is directly responsible for the health of these 2,500 individuals and is therefore financially accountable. No longer will it be sufficient to deal with episodes of care alone and preventive issues only when a person comes into the office. Instead, the doctor and the team must find new ways to interact on an ongoing basis with each person in that population. In practice, this means a major change in how the doctor and the doctor's office (or a group of doctors and their group's team) functions.

Our hypothetical doctor, with a population of patients, will need to interact differently than in the past. This represents new work, and much of the work should be delegated to team members. For example, the 5 percent of the population with multiple chronic diseases needs close care coordination. This means frequent checks that the patient is actually taking medications as prescribed, that blood sugar levels of diabetic patients are under control, that visits to specialists are arranged effectively, and that the specialist's recommendations are addressed in a timely fashion. All of this may require new skills and techniques, which will require new training of nurses and other staff in the office. It will also require collaboration with the PCP. As part of this collaboration, organizing the office to complete these tasks substantially reduces the risk of a malpractice suit, if only because decisions are implemented rather than lost in the shuffle.

For the many patients who are overweight and at high risk for developing diabetes, the team should be in contact with them, offering weight reduction assistance and nutrition counseling. In addition, the team must understand the person's underlying culture, family setting and psychology that drives the weight gain. This is work that most nurses and doctors are not well-trained to do. It requires education about the methods and techniques used to change the thought processes that are the patients' underlying drivers of adverse behaviors. Since these are likely individuals who do not frequent the doctor's office, it is the team's responsibility to reach out proactively – a distinct change from the past that is both disruptive and transformational.

In addition, the doctor's office itself likely requires new infrastructure. Your doctor may have an electronic health record (EHR) in place, but these EHRs were designed to assist with episodic health care, not population health concepts. Either the electronic health record must be updated, or other computerized methods will be required to assist the doctor and the team with the types of alerts that are required for effective population health management.

Another big change includes converting the office staff from a group that assists the doctor and the doctor's needs to one that focuses on the patient's needs. This is another disruptive and transformational change. But if the doctor is to be effective in the new model of accountability for population health care, these changes will occur out of necessity because the practice will only be paid for measurable outcomes.

I have written here about population health from the PCPs' vantage. But there are many "players" that can and will affect a population's health, among them are the local health department, the local community hospital, the various insurers, and of course the individuals themselves. If you accept that the PCP is and should be the center point/the backbone of the health-care system, then the PCP should be the catalyst among these many that are critical to affecting change. Sans that, population health becomes a set of multiple definitions with varied individuals and organizations in search of coordination of purpose and execution. For example, reliance on population health data is clearly important which means there needs to be a good level of harmony between/among the health department, the hospital and the insurance organizations. The PCP becomes the logical center piece for influencing what questions are asked, what is collected and what is measured and for what purpose. And, in the end, remembering that population health is all about the health of each individual.

As in so many situations, the perception of what needs to be done often depends which part of the elephant you touch. Not everyone has a PCP. If the population is in a socioeconomically-deprived urban or rural area with no particular focus of healthcare, the needs and the processes to solve the problems will be much different. In whatever setting, one absolute key factor is the payment system. How is it structured? What are the incentives? Will it be more of the same with added requirements and paperwork, or will it be designed around population health in a way that allows the team – doctor, nurse, NP, PA, others – to get the job done?

My personal concern is that policymakers, self-appointed health care gurus and payers who have never held a stethoscope, taken a patient's history, or walked the halls of a hospital at night, will look to the primary care physician to take on a larger population rather than a smaller population. Their rationale will be that the electronic health records, other software assists, a well-organized functioning team and a new approach to care will, all combined, allow the physician and office team to care for a larger population of individuals. To some degree, they will be correct. But no amount of software or other staff can offer the caring, humanism and healing that comes from a PCP who has time to listen and think.

CHAPTER NINE

WHY PRIMARY CARE PHYSICIANS ARE SO FED UP (AND WHY YOU SHOULD CARE)

To say that PCPs are frustrated is a gross understatement. This frustration provides the motivation to close their private practices. My interviews have brought out strong comments. Here are a few followed by comments on specific issues:

"I felt like a hamster on a wheel. Patients want time and I could not give it to them. I was in a failed profession."

"I was charged [by the HMO employer] with 2,200 patients, mostly sick patients, and I was paid $120,000. That's too many patients at any price; I had to see about 20 per day. I couldn't get them seen and do all the documentation except during my 'family' time. I crawled into bed exhausted with 'nothing left,' yet it started again tomorrow morning. I had nothing left for me – or my husband and children." [She quit and went back to school for an MBA and a career change.]

"Most people just do not understand the role or the value of the PCP. But we have not been as effective as we should be – if we only had fewer patients each to care for. There is a deep divide between the average person and us PCPs. Do we understand each other? Do we listen to each other? Do we know each other's frustrations and even anger? Or do we just think about ourselves and feel even more frustrated that we seem unable to do anything constructive about it?"

"I feel a lack of respect, of appreciation despite all I do for my patients. People just don't realize what we PCPs can and do for their health. Yet I have no time with them. It is really frustrating. It makes me angry."

"If you haven't walked the life, you just cannot understand it. I and my colleagues carry a lot of responsibility, and we keep it with us all the time, in the shower, eating dinner, falling asleep. I am worrying about your health, not just when I see you in the office."

"I was rising up the leadership levels of our professional society, but I came to realize that it just did not and would not likely address the needs of the PCP. So I opted out of further involvement. It was not worth it."

Dr. Daniela Drake wrote an article for The Daily Beast that "went viral" entitled "How being a doctor became the most miserable profession." Here is an excerpt.

"Simply put, being a doctor has become a miserable and humiliating undertaking. Indeed, many doctors feel that America has declared war on physicians – and both physicians and patients are the losers.... Unfortunately, things are only getting worse for most doctors, especially those who still accept health insurance... In fact, difficulty dealing with insurers has caused many physicians to close their practices and become employees... But the primary care doctor doesn't have the political power to say no to anything – so the "to-do" list continues to lengthen. A stunning and unmanageable number of forms – often illegible – show up daily on a physician's desk needing to be signed... To be sure, many people with good intentions are working toward solving the healthcare crisis. But the answers they've come up with are driving up costs and driving out doctors."

Survey Results

The "2014 Survey of America's Physicians" had the following major observations: 81% of physicians (not just primary care) feel overextended or at full capacity, up from 76% in 2008. Forty four percent plan to reduce patient access to their practice by a reducing the number of patients seen, retiring, working part time or closing the practice to new patients. This would mean the effective reduction in the physician workforce of "tens of thousands of full time equivalents." Seventy two percent believe there is a shortage of physicians today. There has been a dramatic drop in private practitioners – only 35% are in independent practice in 2014 compared to 49% in 2012 and 62% in 2008. And 53% now describe themselves as employees of a hospital or medical group whereas it was 44% in 2012 and 38% in 2008. Almost one-third would not choose medicine if they could relive their careers today but 50% would still recommend medicine as a career to their children or other young people. Nearly 70% reported that their autonomy has been greatly diminished.[40]

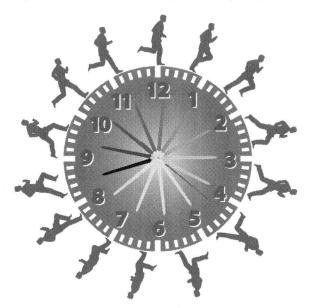

The "Medscape Internist Lifestyle Report 2015" found that 50% of general internists and 50% of family medicine physicians are burned out, defined as "loss of enthusiasm for work, feelings of cynicism and low sense of personal accomplishment." Of those internists who reported burnout, they rated its intensity at 4.8 on a scale of 1 to 7 where 1 – "does not interfere with my life" and 7 – "so severe that I am thinking of leaving medicine." The top five reasons given in rank order were: bureaucratic tasks, too many hours at work, income not high enough, feeling like a cog in the wheel and increasing computerization of practice.[41]

Lack of Time

In my interviews, PCPs stated that their greatest frustration is "time, time, time." Every PCP said that time – or lack of time – was the greatest frustration of their practice. Or if they now were in a practice that limited the patient number to a manageable level, time was the greatest frustration previously.

Each knew that they could not give the time needed to provide the level of care that they were capable of giving and that their patients deserved.

Stated somewhat differently, they said it was frustrating to always focus on meeting overhead costs and earn what they thought was a reasonable income. To do so meant less time with patients, a sense of frustration and perhaps even guilt. New practice patterns have meant not being readily available to patients, not visiting them at the hospital or ER, and no longer effectively being the "captain of the ship."

Time is important to listen to you and it is important for a chance to think about what you said. We often do not stop to appreciate that thinking is an important function and thinking takes time. As an analogy, for those of you who follow *The Big Bang Theory* comedy on TV, a friend directed me to the episode where two physicists say to each other "It's time to get to work." The next scene is the two of them staring at a problem-filled erase board to the tune "The Eye of the Tiger." It then cuts to them in different poses, still staring at the board.[42] It is funny but it is also accurate in that a good percentage of their "work" is thinking about a problem. A concept difficult for many of us to grasp since our culture encourages "doing" and views contemplation as "doing nothing."

Employed PCPs often complain about lack of time, just as those in private practice. A Medscape survey found that 41 percent had no daily quota, but 22 percent were expected to see 16-20 patients per day; 22 percent were expected to see 21-25 per day and 5 percent had a quota of 26-30 patient visits each day.

A physician in an academic medical center wrote: "As you know, practicing good medicine in the US has become challenging; we are supposed to see follow-up patients in 15 min slots including numerous irrelevant EHR clicks (with my back now turned toward the patient) and dropping the bill within the 15 minute slot! The typical referral note I receive is 7-10 pages long but it says little about what the patient's problems are. I am not considered a "productive faculty" member because I take 30-45 minutes per patient visit and I do not write my note until after the visit ...notes I am told are "unconventional" because I start with one page maximum of the basics of the patient's status and then I do the 7-8 pages of clicking to drop the bill. Very sad."

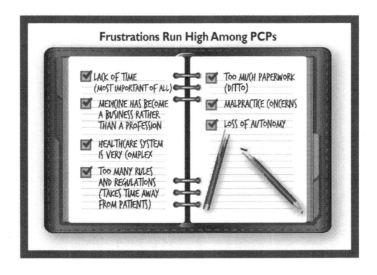

Medicine Has Become a Business

In other words, PCPs believe the practice of medicine has become a business rather than an honored profession. We all recognize that pharmaceutical companies aim to profit, as do the medical device companies, diagnostics firms and for-profit insurers. Of course the doctor wants to earn a good income. Nevertheless, many feel the needs of running the business side of the practice have not only limited the time available but also have compromised the ethics and professionalism that should be the bedrock of being a physician. "No money, no mission," they say, but mission has been compromised.

As Art Caplan PhD, director of medical ethics at New York University Medical Center said in a Medscape survey, "Medicine has become a business, with too much emphasis on business practices and not enough on ethics and professionalism."[43] And primary care physician Dr. Steven Horvitz suggested, "The healthcare system is changing. It is becoming a corporate- and government-controlled system. If that is what makes you comfortable you will get utmost satisfaction from being a physician. If you do not like the corporate world, beware, and develop a good business plan to allow yourself to succeed on your own."

Complexity

Another common frustration refrain is the complexity of the healthcare delivery system. Nothing is ever simple to accomplish. As one of the interviewees said to me about the fragmented system, "I need to go an extra mile to communicate with my patients but there is not enough time to do it."

Frustrations with Requirements and Regulations

PCPs believe that there are a "fearsome" number of rules, regulations and guidelines that must be followed to run a practice. Each may have been initiated with good intentions, but each adds to the workload of the doctor and the practice team, often without any apparent improvement in care. All agree that there must be guidelines, but all also state that the current guidelines need a careful review with elimination of those that do not offer measurable quality improvement. A few of these will be discussed below.

In the Medscape survey referred to previously, Dr. Paul Auwaeter of Johns Hopkins said, "My biggest complaint: The tyranny of excellence. What I mean by this is the fearsome number of rules, regulations and suggestions/guidelines that all may be well intentioned but which now comprise a growing amount of clinicians' time. A careful analysis of those that truly offer significant benefit, and removal of those with lower impact, would be a boon to clinicians."[36]

Frustrations with Insurers

Whether referring to Medicare, Medicaid or commercial insurers, PCPs complain that they are not adequately reimbursed for cognitive services. This is the root cause of the crisis in primary care, and they note that until this is corrected, the crisis will persist and worsen, with fewer medical school graduates electing to enter primary care.

Dr. Steven Horvitz expressed the issue as, "Third-party insurance and government interference need to be greatly reduced so that physicians can do their jobs without having our hands tied behind our backs." His is a common refrain of PCPs, indeed all physicians. "The biggest barrier to practicing medicine today is the third-party interference, whether it be from health insurers such as HMOs and PPOs or government regulations and mandates such as EMRs and HIPAA. A physician's No. 1 priority must be the patient sitting across the table. But with third parties whispering in your ears about this formulary or that pre-certification, it makes it difficult to focus solely on the patient."[44]

A common refrain in my PCP interviews was that commercial insurers are difficult, frustrating to deal with, and take an increasingly large amount of time to get preauthorization for a test or settle issues related to billing. Simply being on hold is sometimes the greatest frustration. Each practice must hire staff to interact with insurers. If the administrative assistant cannot get the authorization, as is often the case, then the PCP must make the call and try to get to a higher level for approval. Usually the insurer will consent if the PCP is diligent and persistent, but the time wasted is "enormous."

An individual who works in a doctor's office offered this comment: "Having seen this in action numerous times working for Dr. McMullen, I've cynically come to believe that the insurance companies want the doctor to give up pursuing the scan, so they make authorization for it as difficult, frustrating and time consuming as it can be. I don't think most patients understand the huge amount of time doctors are often forced to spend just trying to get their decision covered by patient insurance. Perhaps if they did, there would be more outrage and lobbying to change it."

Contrast that statement with a comment from a former board member of a large health insurance company: "We learned that despite having a bevy of doctors and nurses field calls for authorization, our savings were miniscule. Hardly worth the effort and certainly we engendered a lot of hard feelings from our physicians."

Other frustrations include trying to determine what drugs are covered on an individual insurer's formulary (each insurer's formulary is different) and dealing with the reimbursement methodology for each individual. Some insurers are slow to pay reimbursements, which means the doctor must carry high working capital. That is difficult for a small practice.

More than one PCP noted the amount of time required to arrange for services such as home care, which, if the insurer was logical, would actually prevent additional expensive time in the ER, doctor's office or hospital. PCPs find it exceedingly frustrating to deal with non-medical people at the insurance company who deny tests or medications that the doctors feel are in the patient's best interest.

PCPs feel at the mercy of insurers. "The [commercial] insurer presents you with a contract which outlines its reimbursement levels (usually at some percent of Medicare rates) and the policies and procedures that the PCP has to follow. You basically have to sign. There is no negotiation possible," one said. That is one reason why PCPs are leaving private practice and joining the local hospital as an employee. The hospital is large enough to negotiate a somewhat larger fee schedule.

PCPs find it frustrating that they need to learn the differences among insurers – different formularies, approval requirements and reimbursements for different services. It is one more time sink that does nothing to help the patient receive quality care. Most PCPs (and probably most all other physicians) see insurers as faceless bureaucracies. As one interviewee told me, "Commercial insurance and Medicare are both moving targets. You can be the best free throw shooter in the game, but as soon as you release the ball, they move the basket. Coding changes, so many claims get returned because a CPT billing or ICD-9 code has changed. [CPT and ICD-9 are systems used in the billing and coding process for physician and hospital reimbursement.] We are often never notified of these changes. Or if they do, we are so inundated in paperwork that you can't keep your eye on the ball. Medicare requires even more paperwork to be filled out by the PCP at our expense without any compensation."

One PCP reported that he and his partners decided to no longer accept United Health Care insurance from their patients and they were close to refusing Aetna. The companies had become too burdensome. Fortunately for their patients with Aetna, the company improved substantially.

Another PCP interviewee used his driving time to make calls to insurers to get preauthorizations. Since they need to be called for "everything," using drive time did not interfere with his practice time, although it did mean losing time for "just listening to the radio and chilling out for a few minutes at the end of the day. I call an 800 number, push 7 buttons, and get asked, 'what is the patient's insurance number?' Fair enough, but then they want his date of birth, my practice identification number with their company, and more. I am trying to help the patient, but the insurer makes me go through hoops. It is very frustrating." Another said, "I only order something if I really think the patient needs it. But I have to deal with a paper pusher with much less knowledge than me to get approval. It is demeaning to me."

Of course, insurers have a contrary perspective of claims forms improperly completed and preauthorization requests made without supporting evidence. The truth is certainly somewhere in between, with both doctors and insurers frustrated.

A recent study of family physicians' perceptions of the documentation and billing rules for Medicare, Medicaid and commercial insurance found the "documentation and coding rules and common fees for procedures and preventive services were reasonable." But "the documentation rules for all other visit types were perceived as unnecessarily complicated and unclear. The existing codes did not describe the actual work for common clinic visits....inadequate payment for complex patients...services requiring extra time beyond a standard office visit, non-face-to-face time, and others. The rules created unintended negative consequences, such as family physicians not accepting Medicare or Medicaid patients, inaccurate documentation, poor-quality care, and system inefficiencies such as unnecessary tests and referrals...Family physicians expressed many problems and frustrations with the documentation, coding and billing rules and felt the system undervalued and unappreciated them for the complex and comprehensive care they provide. Altogether, the typical PCP spends about one hour of his or her own time on insurance paperwork and phone calls per day."[45]

Frustrations with Government

Government regulations are also a major cause of physician frustration. They create serious constraints and often cause higher costs. The PCPs I interviewed said HIPAA [referring to the health care portability act that, among other things, was designed to assure protection of confidentiality with patient health information] regulations are a fundamentally good idea but are often implemented in a manner that impedes good care. For example, a PCP treated a patient with a crushed foot. She was sent to the local trauma center, and when he called to follow-up, he was told, "Can't discuss it with you; HIPAA regs."

Although not a PCP, the president of the Erie County Medical Society said in his inaugural address, "Our nation does not treat our doctors as the invaluable resource they are. Specifically, to what extent have our federal and state governments, their bureaucracies and policies harmed our doctors and our nation's medical system? .... The two basic assumptions governments make which cause harm to the medical profession, and thus ultimately harm patients, are that they know better than you do, doctor, and that they should tell you what to do. Governments are literally gravely wrong in using these assumptions as the basis for over-regulation. ... Thus notions about documentation spawn a high volume of 'make work' which has no contribution to patient outcomes. *Doctors and nurses today spend half of their working time not on patients, but on producing documentation.* [His italics] Even with that, insurers widely abuse documentation excuses to not pay doctors and hospitals. Keeping reasonable records in some understandable form is necessary, but documentation has become a false god, and ... the government must stop forcing you to serve it. You should be serving the patient."[46]

Dr. Andy Lazris writes eloquently about frustrations with Medicare in particular in his book *Curing Medicare.*

In these statements about insurers and government, the underlying frustration and anger is due to a loss of autonomy. Listen carefully to your own PCP (or specialist) and ask about autonomy.

The Electronic Medical Record

The following from Dr. Henry Black of New York University Medical Center neatly sums up what a lot of physicians feel about the electronic medical record. "The imposition of computers between the doctor and the patient has almost ruined that interaction...all we get is doctors staring into computers rather than patients' faces...The one I was using was apparently designed by payers to improve billing and collections, not by doctors to improve patient care."[36]

Another common complaint, closely related to frustration with government, is the requirement to have a functioning electronic health record, or EHR, or otherwise face penalties and lower Medicare reimbursements. The following comment is representative of what many PCPs told me: "The EHR really slows me down. It should be the other way around. It is great to find a report but time consuming to do data entry. If I put in the data as we are talking, then I am not really focused on the patient but on the computer screen. That is not an advance; it is a big loss." Others said they "feel like a clerk. It is not designed for how a doctor works." This last comment has been near universal for at least a decade despite newer EHRs. In many hospital settings, the physicians vote with their feet – that is, they write in the chart or dictate notes like they always have and send them into the EHR when they return from the pool. That's OK, but it does not align with the concept of having the data available in real time and at any location.

The EHR creates another problem. During short visits, the doctor often inputs the history and physical examination findings as he or she proceeds. This means the doctor does not make eye contact with you, disrupting the easy flow of conversation that is essential to good diagnosis and critical to healing.

An additional problem with the EHR is the way information is entered. In cognitive (as opposed to procedural) physician practices, such as with a PCP, the history is critical. But many EHRs are designed to use drop-down boxes and checkmarks. These lose the nuances of the history that can only be recorded in prose.

Finally, most PCPs stated that the EHR slowed them down initially and substantially. The learning curve was steep and the EHR was not intuitive to learn. The system not only cost high dollars to purchase, but it cost many dollars in lost productivity for many months. Some felt it continued to be a "drag" on their practice work indefinitely. One said, "Just one more government requirement that slows me down and interferes with my patient relationships."

A recent survey by MPI Group for Medical Economics found that nearly half of physicians believe EHRs are actually making patient care worse, with 23 percent saying it is significantly worse. Plus, the government incentives are not enough to pay for the unanticipated costs, including adding more staff and a loss of physician productivity – the exact problems the EHR was intended to decrease, along with improving patient care. Among other observations, two thirds said they dislike the functionality of the system, and nearly 70 percent said it has not helped coordination of care with hospitals (another big driver of why the EHR was supposed to add value). In addition, about one-half believe they cost too much.

A common refrain among PCPs that I have interviewed is that the EHR is fundamentally designed for billing and coding purposes. But the original – and still fundamental – purpose of a patient's chart has always been to record observations that would be useful to the doctor later or for another provider to understand. To most PCPs, that purpose is no longer front and center.

This is not a pretty picture of a technology that was supposed to make care better, reduce costs and increase physician productivity. Presumably, this survey is representative, meaning that respondents were not only the disillusioned. Regardless, there is real work to be done before the EHR will be seen as a boon to the primary care physician. This is unlike the hospital experience where, despite many grumblings, doctors tend to find the EHR useful, especially for ordering a test or imaging procedure or receiving an alert about a medication or test result. But just as in the office setting, many internists and primary care physicians indicate that writing progress notes about their patients in the hospital electronic medical record is fraught with frustrations.

Other Frustrations

Important information is lost during the limited communication that occurs when a patient is discharged from a hospital to home or nursing home. Often the PCP does not know that a patient was hospitalized until they show up for the next appointment in the office. This is an indictment of the entire American health care delivery system.

Concern about malpractice litigation is another important issue, driving a need to practice defensive medicine with its associated increased costs. Malpractice suits are generally less common among primary care practitioners than among specialists. However, PCPs tend to be anxious and practice defensively, meaning more tests and more specialist referrals. Interestingly, when the actual data are analyzed, the most common suits, nearly 75 percent, relate to delayed diagnosis or missed diagnosis, according to a study in the

Journal of the American Medical Association.[47] The authors suggest that, in most cases, it was the result of breakdowns in office processes – not updating a patient's record with new information, not following through with the PCP's request for a test or referral, or not actively following up with a patient once results were returned. The problem, as I understand it, is less a need for "defensive medicine" but rather a need to work on internal office workflow, complete with built-in checks to ensure that the "ball is not dropped" by doctors or staff. Look back to the discussion about accountable care organizations and population health and how those models could actually reduce the risk of malpractice as a result of better care quality and better office organization.

Loss of Autonomy

During interviews with PCPs, "loss of autonomy" was stated in many forms, but the message was clear. PCPs cannot make the decisions, as in the past, about what is in the best interest of you, the patient. (Look back on the story that begins Chapter 1. Dr. Foster was denied obtaining an MRI for his patient. If he had not insisted and persisted, the end result would have been negative for the patient's future health). They cannot take time with you, order a test or image without permission, or give a prescription without approval. This is the essence of the PCPs' frustrations. One said, "I cannot be the physician I was trained to be or know I could and should be for my patients."

Consider this analogy from PCP Dr. Jordan Grumet, who maintains a blog about primary care.[48] He was driving one day and saw a man on a bicycle wearing no helmet. He was using earphones and listening to music. He was darting in and out of traffic but was not holding the handlebars; instead, he was holding a book. Multi-tasking taken to the limits. But is it safe? Dr. Grumet compares this to evaluating a sick patient while concurrently having to meet meaningful use of the EHR, follow checklists, abide by HIPAA standards and fill out innumerable insurance forms. Is this multi-tasking, he asks, or is it just distraction leading to less adequate care?

CHAPTER TEN
WHY PATIENTS ARE LOSING PATIENCE

"The patient will no longer be patient" is an apt expression for the changing nature of a patient's expectation with his or her doctor. In prior generations, the expectation was that the doctor was not to be questioned, that he or she knew what was right, that long waits were part of the experience, and that patients were not educated enough to understand their medical problems. Just do as the doctor says. That is no longer the case.

Call them patients, clients or consumers. By whatever name, they (that means you) do not like the current healthcare delivery system. You may like your doctor on a personal basis but are nevertheless frustrated that it takes an average of 20.5 days to be seen by the physician. You are also frustrated that you frequently sit in the waiting room for a protracted time, get only a few minutes of actual "face time" with your doctor, are not fully listened to or understood, and are not fully informed about what the doctor was thinking or why a certain test or prescription was ordered. Furthermore, you may have realized that you are not really the doctor's customer since the insurance company tells the doctor if and how much he or she can receive as a reimbursement for your care. And you are not the insurer's customer either. Your employer is or the government (through Medicare or Medicaid) is really the customer of the insurer since they pay the insurers' bills.

But "consumerism" is growing, and more patients are taking steps to take charge. Their needs and wants are becoming clear, and more patients like you are insisting that they be considered the customer. To repeat the apt phrase: "The patient will no longer be patient."

Today, patients are insisting on short wait times, expecting the doctor's office to notify them if the doctor is running late – perhaps by a text message – so they can come in later than scheduled, asking for email connection with the physician as appropriate, and expecting that the physician will take the time to close the information gap between them.

Patients want and expect respect, as shown by all of the service issues listed above, a professional demeanor, assurance of confidentiality, and of course, high quality care with an assurance of safety. It is the Golden Rule – you want your physician to treat you the way he or she would want to be treated.

Absent respect, as judged and perceived by you, it is not unusual today for the patient to look elsewhere for care. This is a real change. Patients are becoming consumers and acting like it.

General Expectations

A recent survey done by the Cleveland Clinic found that the most aggravating issues for patients were long waits at the office, a lack of empathy and a sense of rushed appointments. They would like to sense empathy, be listened to and feel respected. They would also appreciate being able to contact the physician directly.[49]

Listening – and listening deeper and longer – is the first request by the patient of the PCP. Of course, this is often a silent request. But you want your doctor to care about you and how you feel, not just focus on the symptom or disease at hand. Sometimes we do not appreciate what underlying factors might have prompted our problem, and we need the doctor to search and help us find it. As part of listening, you want and prefer good eye contact, a pleasant and nonjudgmental conversation, and an opportunity to express your issues in your own words, at your own pace, and perhaps with appropriate prompting from the physician. This requires that the physician is attuned to you during this critical period of interaction. Computers are great, but they can interfere if the doctor is focused on it instead of you.

A 2014 study by the Associated Press and NORC [Nutrition and Obesity Research Center of the University of Chicago, which now does many health-related projects other than its namesake objective] put a light on how "Americans Evaluate Provider Quality." Bottom line – patients are most focused on their relationship with their doctor, which is what I have referred to as "relationship medicine." Listening, being attentive and interested, and relating to the patient were at the top of the list of characteristics important to patients. Education, experience and the office environment were at the bottom. When asked about the factor that makes for a poor quality doctor, the top answers included: doesn't listen, not attentive, and lack of time with patients. When judging the location of high-quality care, the rank order was doctor's offices, hospitals, emergency rooms, retail clinics like Wal-Mart and Walgreens and walk-in clinics or urgent care centers. For trustworthy information about quality locations and doctors, respondents turned to family members and friends (62 percent) and their regular health care provider (47 percent) but not to federal and state agencies (17 percent), free web sites like Yelp or paid ratings sites like Angie's List (10-11 percent) or newspapers and magazines (6 percent). As summarized by the authors, "When it comes to what being a quality health care provider means, there is a disconnect between how experts and consumers define it. Most Americans focus on the doctor-patient *relationship* [my italics] and interactions in the doctor's office, with fewer thinking about the effectiveness of treatments or their own health outcomes. Further, individuals report that they value provider quality over cost and are willing to pay more for higher-quality doctors."[50]

As Dr. Pamela Wible, a family physician, expressed it – "Listen up, docs: Patients just want the real you. Ya know—YOU. The competent and caring you who really listens with compassion. The real you that talks like a real person and answers people with the honest truth in words they understand. The you that treats patients like family. Does it matter if you've got glitter on your eyelids? Or if you come in after hours in sweatpants? Or if your kid tags along with you to work? Actually patients think those things are kinda cool. So how do I know what patients want? *I ask them.* [my italics] And what they want more than anything else is a doctor who is courageous enough to be real."[51]

Use of Social Media

Patients use the Internet more than any other source for health information – for better or worse, evidence-based or not. They also use it to connect and communicate with family and friends regarding health issues and with groups or communities of others who have the same illness. To a lesser degree, they use it to communicate with their healthcare providers.

Patients increasingly use social media to talk to each other. They join or create information exchanges about rare or terrifying diseases. They develop virtual support groups to learn how others handle the rigors of cancer chemotherapy, the loss of hair, the fatigue and the isolation. Perhaps most significantly, patients rate their doctors and hospitals via social media. The old adage that a "happy customer will tell someone but an unhappy one will tell 10 others" is magnified logarithmically with social media. Increasingly, patients expect their physicians, nurse practitioners and other providers to communicate digitally. They expect email for sure, texting more and sometimes via Skype or other telemedicine techniques. This can save a visit to the office or prevent a trip to the ER, but as noted earlier, social media is still rarely used by PCPs, at least by the PCPs I interviewed. There is no reason why you should not have similar expectations of your physician – but you may need to be prepared to pay for it.

Public Reporting and Patient Empowerment

Although largely driven by government rather than the general public, there is a growing consensus in favor of public reporting of outcomes. Most outcome measures are of interest to academics and others in the healthcare arena but seem to be of limited interest to patients. Polls show that few individuals make use of the available information, perhaps because it is not seen as that relevant to their concerns. Knowing a surgeon's complication rate is of interest if it is outside the range of others, but minor differences are not likely relevant to a decision. But other factors may be of greater importance. The more important question for a patient – which is not easily available – is whether a proposed course of action is the best option. The answer might include not only medical evidence but also what it will cost out of pocket given the individual's insurance coverage and what he or she can expect as a result of the drug, procedure or behavior modification. Will the disease/condition be improved? By how much? What about side effects and relative costs of one approach versus another? Current public reporting systems are not designed with these types of questions in mind.

Payment Expectations

As insurance has morphed from the concept of "major medical" or catastrophic care to today's prepaid medical care, most people have come to expect their insurance to pay for everything. Co-pays and deductibles have been added and increased as total medical care costs have risen. Employers expect employees to pay a greater percentage of premiums and use co-pays and deductibles to dissuade trips to the doctor. But we, as patients, are not accustomed to having our doctor charge for "extras" such as using email, Skype or even a phone consultation. One patient expressed this sentiment: "The few times I've had to deal with lawyers, they charged for every interaction. Every phone call and email. People expect it. Can you imagine the outcry if doctors tried the same thing? I'd be willing to pay a reduced out-of-pocket fee for a 'phone consult' to avoid going to the office if there was a very routine problem. Again, lawyers charge for every interaction, but they charge less for a phone conversation as opposed to going to the office. " It is not our expectation now, but this will change, I suspect, because payment for medical care is changing.

Complementary Medicine Expectations

Complementary medicine is commonplace and growing, including acupuncture, massage, various mind-body approaches, herbal remedies and chiropractic services. Many have stood the test of time, and some have now been shown by solid research to be effective. Some reports indicate that more money is spent on complementary medicine practitioners than on primary care. But PCPs are often not aware that the patient has been to a complementary medicine practitioner. One patient said, "I'm always hesitant to tell a doctor about the supplements I take and when I do, I brace myself for the eye roll or lecture about their ineffectiveness. No one has ever engaged me in a discussion about nutrition, despite my attempts, obvious interest and knowledge base." This comes from a medically knowledgeable person, yet he is uncomfortable sharing these thoughts with his PCP. As many of the PCPs explained in the interviews, they realize their patients frequent alternative providers. Interestingly, in this case it was not "alternative" medicine but commonly used over-the-counter supplements that he took. Still, there is not enough communication between PCPs and patients about "extra-medical" treatments and medications.

One Physician's Observations of his New Primary Care Doctor

Dr. Feldman worked as a specialist in a large university hospital about 25 miles from his home throughout his career. He was healthy and had no primary care physician but would go to whichever staff member seemed pertinent when he had an occasional problem. His wife saw her gynecologist annually. Now, both retired, they decided it was time to develop a relationship with a PCP near to home. After checking with some friends and neighbors, they settled on a respected, relatively young PCP. Feldman brought a typed two-page sheet with him, outlining his past medical history, few medications, vitamins and supplements. He filled out pages of paperwork as a first-time patient. Blood was drawn for a general screening, and the results would be available when he met with the doctor a few days later. Dr. Feldman questioned the decision to draw blood work before the doctor got to know him or do a history or exam. He wondered, "Wouldn't it be better to then decide what blood work might be appropriate?" He found the doctor pleasant but difficult to engage. The doctor sat with his computer on his lap and entered information as they discussed Dr. Feldman's history. There was little eye contact. "I know that it interferes with our interaction, but I need to input all this information, so I really need to do it now rather than later," the doctor said. "There is just so much time."

From this and other comments, it was obvious that the doctor was on a tight schedule. He was friendly and engaged but with no idle conversation and no questions that would enhance his knowledge about Dr. Feldman's family or social setting. I asked him if he would stick with the young doctor. "Yes, I liked him despite the abruptness of the encounter. And although I disagree with the decision about blood work before knowing what might be appropriate, I have to admit that he picked up hypothyroidism (a thyroid that is not producing normal amounts of thyroid hormone) in my wife with his screening test. In retrospect, she had some telltale clues, but we both had just ascribed them to getting older. Now she feels much better on proper medication. Of course, he would have figured this out anyway because it would have been part of his testing later."

The message: Patients are beginning to act like the consumers they are in other venues. They want to be heard, have time with their doctor, develop a close relationship, and sense trust. The patient will simply no longer be "patient." Doctors need to grasp this fundamental expectation and be responsive – or lose trust and business.

PART III

THE CHANGING NATURE OF ILLNESSES: FROM ACUTE TO CHRONIC

Unlike the devastating infectious diseases of a century ago, such as pneumonia and typhoid, today's most common diseases are chronic: heart and lung disease, diabetes and cancer. Some are due to aging, but most are due to adverse lifestyles and behaviors over many years. They are expensive to treat since they persist for life in most cases. Chronic disease treatment requires a different approach to care that demands time-consuming attention and often the assistance of a team of providers who manage different symptoms and medications. The primary care physician can be the critical link to both preventing these illnesses and treating them effectively when they develop.

Chapter Eleven
THE IMPACT OF CHRONIC DISEASES

The diseases that a physician sees today are markedly different than in years past. Decades ago, most illnesses were acute (or temporary, such as pneumonia and appendicitis) but today the vast majority are chronic that stick with us for life. This is a critical transition that dramatically affects how the PCP conducts his or her practice. What is this transition and how did it occur?

Chronic disease is transforming health, medical costs and the delivery of care. Diseases such as diabetes, heart failure, emphysema, and cancer are chronic. Once developed, they usually last a lifetime, are difficult to manage and expensive to treat. Chronic illnesses, once rare, are becoming commonplace. They are responsible for the vast majority of health care costs but are to a large degree preventable. The PCP could be a major factor in restricting the development of these diseases, but most do not do so effectively due to a lack of time. The PCP can manage chronic illnesses, for the most part, and provide careful coordination when referrals are needed. But this intense attention and coordination is not the norm. The reason, as you will recognize, is lack of time, not lack of skill or interest on the part of the PCP.

Chronic illnesses have two primary antecedents – aging and adverse behaviors. There has been a fairly remarkable increase in average lifespans and an increasing percentage of those who live a longer time. With aging comes certain impairments, including impaired vision, hearing, mobility (osteoarthritis), bone strength (osteoporosis with fractures), dentition (and with it impaired nutrition) and cognition (including Alzheimer's). Many of these are partially preventable. Good diet and exercise limit osteoporosis and joint damage, dental hygiene limits loss of teeth, avoidance of excessive noise can lessen hearing loss, avoidance of excessive ultraviolet rays from the sun can limit the development of cataracts, and physical and mental exercise can stave off cognition decline for some time. But as we age, many of these impairments, even with excellent self-care, will develop to a small degree and then progress over time.

Adverse behaviors are by far the major cause of most chronic illnesses. McGinnis and Foege analyzed data from 1990 to determine the actual causes of death – not the disease but the antecedent to that disease. About one-half of all deaths were traceable to lifestyle issues. This table shows the highlights.[52]

ACTUAL CAUSES OF DEATH IN THE UNITED STATES - 1990	
Tobacco	400,000
Diet and Activity	300,000
Alcohol	100,000
Microbial Agents	90,000
Toxic Agents	60,000
Firearms	35,000
Sexual Behaviors	30,000
Motor Vehicles	25,000
Illicit Drugs	20,000

The Evolution of Chronic Disease in Modern Society

In 1900, the three most common causes of death in the U.S. were typhoid, tuberculosis and pneumonia – all infectious diseases. In 2010, the three most common causes of death in the U.S. were cardiovascular, cancer and lung disease – all chronic illnesses, mostly lifestyle-related and all largely preventable. (The Figure is an adaption from Jones, et al in *The New England Journal of Medicine*[53]) Not surprisingly, obesity and obesity-related diabetes have also emerged as major predisposing factors to chronic illness and are climbing the list of primary causes of death. In addition, the presence of Alzheimer's and suicide among the common primary causes of death today illustrates the complexity of how aging and mental health are impacting illness and survival. They further signal the reality that mental health has become an entirely new segment of concern in the ever growing list of chronic diseases in our society. The most important underlying drivers of these chronic illnesses, according to a Centers for Disease Control and Prevention (CDC) report in the *Journal of the American Medical Association,* are tobacco use, poor dietary habits, lack of exercise and alcohol abuse – all modifiable behaviors.[54]

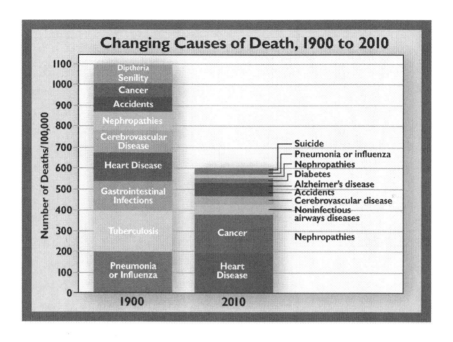

The striking reduction of acute, infectious diseases is a testament to the successful collaboration of both science and society in its development and adoption of sanitation, safe water and food, hygiene, antibiotics and immunizations during the last 100 years. Plus, safer work environments mean less trauma and injury. The trend toward prolonged, chronic diseases now poses a new commensurate challenge for both science and society.

The magnitude of the task at hand was illustrated by the Milken Institute in their 2007 study *An Unhealthy America: The Economic Burden of Chronic Disease.*[55] They evaluated cancer, diabetes, hypertension, stroke, heart disease, pulmonary conditions and mental disorders. The study noted that nearly one-half of Americans had one or more chronic illnesses and that "each has been linked to behavioral and/or environmental risk factors that broad-based prevention programs could address."

Industry has also recognized that 75 percent of their healthcare costs go to the care of just a few diseases – each chronic and each largely preventable.

Insurers further report that 70-85 percent of paid claims are for chronic illnesses. It has also been reported that 85 percent of Medicare enrollees have at least one chronic illness, while more than 50 percent of enrollees have three or more chronic illnesses that require them to take an average of 5 to 7 prescription medications per day. Those with serious chronic illnesses consume most of the health care expenditures. Among Medicare enrollees, for example, just 5 percent consume 43 percent of the money, most all going to treat chronic illnesses. About 20 percent of these patients have serious heart disease and are over age 85. Another 20 percent have end stage kidney failure, which is covered by Medicare at any age. The average expenditure among this group is $108,000 per person per year while using multiple physicians and about 25 prescriptions.

The Milken study further quantified the cost of chronic illnesses to the U.S. economy at more than $1.1 trillion per year in 2007. Among their findings: 109 million Americans – or one-third – have a chronic illness now, and many have more than one, which totals 162 million with chronic diseases. The annual costs of care today are about $275 billion, and the total economic costs are more than $1 trillion per year in lost productivity and work time. Milken estimates that America is on a track for a 42 percent increase in these chronic diseases by 2023 (as a result of aging and behaviors), which is less than a decade from now. If we do nothing to change the way we care for these patients, the annual cost of medical care will be $790 billion, and the total economic costs will be more than $4 trillion.

But there is also hope in the report. "Assuming modest improvements in preventing and treating disease," they project that in 2023, the U.S. "could avoid 40 million cases of chronic disease; could reduce the economic impact of disease by 27 percent, or $1.1 trillion annually; could increase the nation's GDP by $905 billion linked to productivity gains; could also decrease treatment costs by $218 billion per year. Lower obesity rates alone could produce productivity gains of $254 billion and avoid $60 billion in treatment expenditures per year."

Our medical care system has developed over centuries around the process of diagnosing and treating acute illnesses such as pneumonia, a gall bladder attack or appendicitis. The internist gives an antibiotic for the pneumonia and the patient gets better. The surgeon cuts out the gall bladder or the appendix and the patient is cured. One patient, one doctor. But patients with chronic illnesses need a different approach to care. They need long-term care, not episodic care. They need a doctor that attends to the care of their one or more chronic illnesses with intensity. Often they need the PCP to enlist a multi-disciplinary, team-based approach with the PCP serving as the orchestrator or quarterback managing the myriad physician specialists, tests and procedures to allow for a unified, coordinated care approach. It will take a new style of care and great intensity to help these patients, improve their care and reduce total costs.

The future must include a larger focus on wellness, health promotion and preventive medicine. A shift to a new model of care – one effective for chronic illness rather than acute or episodic illness – will substantially improve quality and patient and physician satisfaction and dramatically reduce costs. It is possible to improve quality care and reduce the costs of care while improving patient satisfaction and reducing provider frustration. This requires a new paradigm in management, incentives and compensation for physicians and new responsibilities and incentives for patients as well. The key to this new paradigm is the primary care provider. He or she is well trained and experienced in chronic disease management. But to do this, we must reduce the number of patients under care by each physician to no more than 500-1,000. At this level, the provider can have the time needed to listen, prevent, diagnose, treat and think. This will reduce the excessive use of specialists, tests and procedures and the reflex to hand out a prescription when a lifestyle change would be both more appropriate and more effective.

Chronic Illnesses and Costs of Care

CareFirst, the Blue Cross/Blue Shield company of Maryland, Delaware, Washington D.C. and northern Virginia, plotted the expenditures for those on their insurance plans under 65 years old. The bar on the left in the Figure (adapted from S Dentzer in Health Affairs[56]) divides individuals into five groups based on their wellness/illness gradient – from green for healthy to red for seriously ill.

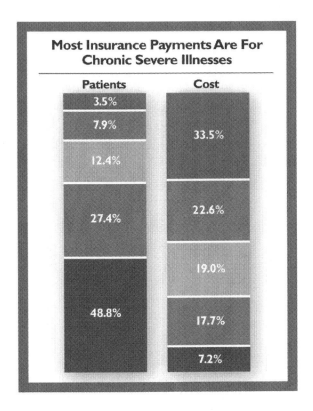

Nearly one-half are well, and a quarter are healthy but with some risk factors. That leaves about 25 percent who have three levels of chronic illnesses. Although only 3.5 percent of individuals have the most serious chronic illnesses, they consume a third of all the money spent for care by CareFirst. Eight percent have a less severe but still serious chronic illness, and these individuals consume nearly a quarter of the dollars. Those with chronic illnesses with limited needs spent another 20 percent. Thus, those with chronic illnesses were responsible for three-quarters of all dollars spent on care.

Aging and Chronic Illnesses

Society is aging rapidly. The number of Americans who are 65 and older will increase by 36 percent to 65 million by 2025. They will represent nearly

20 percent of the total population, compared to about 15 percent today. America will no longer be a "young" country. Those nearing a century are increasing rapidly as well. Today about 576,000 Americans are over 95 years old, and by 2025 the number is expected to increase by about 50 percent to 857,000. Only about 10 percent of the population takes five or more prescription medications, but for those over 65, one-half take four or fewer drugs and the other 50 percent take five or more.[57]

Behaviors and Chronic Illnesses

Older people have more chronic illnesses than younger individuals. But this is not necessarily due to the aging process itself. Yes, older individuals have various impairments, including vision, hearing, mobility and mental capabilities, but the important chronic illnesses such as heart disease, cancer, chronic lung and kidney disease and diabetes are related to long-term effects of lifestyle factors. For example, lung cancer occurs, on average, at age 72, but the steps leading to it began in someone's teens and twenties when smoking began. Heart disease is more common among the elderly, but the process of creating atherosclerosis begins at a young age with the ingestion of the wrong foods, lack of exercise and good dose of chronic stress over a lifetime. Restated, it takes many years for coronary artery plaque to build up sufficient to cause a heart attack. Just because it occurs after age 65 does not imply that it was related to aging. Rather, it just says that the person has lived long enough for the progressive effects of poor and excessive diet, lack of exercise and related obesity, stress and smoking combined with genetic predispositions to finally have the effect of causing overt disease.

Lowering the Costs of Treating Chronic Illnesses

High costs of care are linked to non-transparency in pricing, inappropriate drug advertising, perverse insurance incentives and more. But a few critical elements are largely under the control of each patient and PCP to reverse the high costs of medical care. Personal behavior modification is critical, and your PCP can be helpful here when he or she has the time. For those with chronic illnesses, PCPs can manage the vast majority of issues which means fewer specialist visits, fewer tests and imaging studies, and fewer unnecessary prescriptions – a major savings. The PCP who takes the time to listen and think about your situation also realizes when a symptom has an underlying emotional component that must be addressed. He or she will understand that there is no need for a large battery of tests or referrals.

The first step in this PCP and patient-led change is to engage in effective prevention strategies. We cannot stop aging, though we can slow its progress. Good nutrition, daily moderate exercise, stress modification and no tobacco are the keys to healthy aging and reducing the burden of chronic diseases. Intellectual challenge and social engagement are needed in addition to slow cognitive decline. It is easier said than done, of course, but we need to accept individual responsibility for our own health. We need to understand how our behaviors affect our health in the long-term. Incentives, primarily monetary ones, can have a positive impact. Incentives need to be large enough to be useful yet focused enough to drive someone toward the desired goal. For example, our employer can help with wellness programs to assist us to stop smoking, lose weight, improve our nutrition or deal with stress more effectively. These programs have been proven to work. The financial incentive lowers the employee's portion of their health insurance premium in return for participation, and at the same time it lowers the employer's total costs of healthcare.

The second major step is for our public health system to receive more resources to focus on preventing chronic illnesses with programs aimed at exercise, stress, smoking cessation, use of alcohol in moderation and improved nutrition, each unencumbered by the demands of the tobacco, beverage and food industries. Of course, public health cannot reduce its attention to preventing the major infectious diseases, such as food safety and immunizations, but more resources can help the focus on chronic illnesses as well.

The third major step is to ensure that those with a chronic illness have an excellent PCP who can manage most of the patient's needs but who will also assume an effective care coordination role when necessary. When a patient has a primary care physician who takes the time to fully coordinate all of the elements of care, research shows the use of specialists, tests, procedures and hospitalizations declines, and drug therapy becomes well-managed, often with fewer medications.

When the PCP does have time, the quality of care goes up substantially and the total costs of care come down (detailed in Part Four.) Time spent on prevention will be valuable in the years to come, and time with a difficult diagnostic dilemma will yield the answer without the need for a specialist consult. Plus, time with care coordination will have an immediate effect.

An Issue of Ethical Responsibility

A basic issue that all physicians, including primary care physicians, need to accept and address is how they can personally and specifically help to reduce the costs of medical care. Having time to coordinate care is one important element, but physicians also must accept that they can find various tests, procedures and prescriptions that offer the same advantages as other approaches and cost much less. In the future, the system will focus on "fee for value," so the PCP needs to think differently about use of medical resources. In short, it is no longer possible to have all the data, tests, and specialists' recommendations. Doctors must be somewhat parsimonious – but not to the degree that it diminishes patient care quality.

In an article in the *New England Journal of Medicine*, Dr. Howard Brody argues that physicians, including primary care physicians, need to look carefully at what they do and whether it can stand the test of evidence. He suggests that each specialty, including primary care, establish a "top five" list of the "diagnostic tests or treatments that are very commonly ordered, that are among the most expensive to provide and have been shown by currently available evidence not to provide any meaningful benefit."[58] For example, this might include giving an antibiotic when the patient appears to have a viral infection or ordering thyroid function tests as a routine rather than when the patient expresses a symptom that suggests thyroid dysfunction. The American Society of Clinical Oncology has done an admirable job in addressing this issue with its "Choosing Wisely" program, which describes more than five tests and treatments that should not be used, such as not offering chemotherapy to someone who cannot get into the office without a wheelchair. This example, and others, is based on the idea that those with "poor performance status" rarely respond positively to chemotherapy but will certainly develop side effects.

Chronic illnesses have become common and they account for the vast majority of dollars spent on medical care. In order to achieve a balance of better quality and lower healthcare costs, American medicine needs to focus on individuals at risk and those who already have chronic illnesses. This is where the future of health and wellness lies and where the greatest savings in expenditures resides.

Chapter Twelve
RETHINKING CARE FOR THE CHRONICALLY ILL

In considering how a new model might be organized, it is worth remembering that today America has a medical care system and not a health care system. The focus is on disease once it has occurred, and there is relatively little attention given to maintaining health and wellness.

The new model must create a healthcare system – not just a medical care system. It must recognize the importance of intensive preventive care to maintain wellness. It must address the needs of those with chronic illnesses (who consume 70-85 percent of paid healthcare claims) to both improve quality of care while dramatically reducing the costs of care. It must be redesigned so the patient is the customer that he or she should be – of both the physician and the insurer. It is doable but it means a rethinking of how the delivery system is structured.

Focusing on Chronic Illnesses with Care Coordination

The convergence of lifestyle, demographics and chronic illness will present significant new challenges to the patient, provider, payer and society at large that will change patient care as we know it.

All PCPs in my interviews stated they can – and should – care for most of the issues inherent in those with chronic illnesses. They feel they are well-trained and have the experience and knowledge to provide state-of-the-art care. Most added that they can only do this if they have adequate time, the factor which arises consistently in these discussions.

Each said they can – and do – perform most chronic care themselves and they enjoy doing it. But they were aware that many PCPs have ceded this role to the specialists, where the patient gets "lost in the shuffle." Their favored approach, however, was to save the specialist for the most complex or difficult issues and perhaps for an annual "assessment." Importantly, they recognize the need to "translate" for the patient what the specialist says or proposes. One of their major concerns for their patients is that useful services, such as nutrition, health or fitness coaching, are generally not covered by insurance.

When a patient needs to see a specialist, PCPs believe they should be the "general contractor," or the one who selects the best specialist for the individual patient, often calling to inform the specialist about the reason for the referral and request an early appointment if appropriate.

One PCP who has a concierge practice (see Chapter 14) told me of a patient that arrived in her office one day with the pain of angina. It was snowing outside. The PCP called a cardiologist at a nearby hospital and asked if he could see her promptly. She then actually drove the patient to the cardiologist's office – "I couldn't let her drive in the snow with unstable angina." The patient had a stent placed later that afternoon.

During the interviews, many PCPs said they may send a patient to a diabetes center, for example, on an annual basis for added training about diet, nutrition, insulin education and a general review of their diabetes status. In each case, whether the word was used or not, the PCPs referred to the importance of being the coordinator or quarterback for the patient's care of the chronic illness. Having a good relationship with the patient is important so the patient's progress can be monitored while seeing a specialist. Often the PCP has to "balance the recommendations of the cardiologist versus the pulmonologist versus the endocrinologist who each prescribe medications without regard to the others." It was that lack of care coordination that led Henry (in Chapter 2) to 23 prescription medications but only seven once a PCP took firm control. The interviewees also emphasized that patients with chronic illnesses need to be "listened to," as many of their complications are related to emotional, family or financial issues that need to be discussed for successful treatment. They also stated that they need time with the patient to help them understand that the body is the chief "healer," with medications and other treatments as only adjuncts or assistants to the body's own healing processes.

Here is another story about the importance of time and the need for the PCP to coordinate what each specialist is doing. After I retired, I was asked if I would talk to Mrs. Bennett. She had lost her sense of taste recently. Her PCP had no idea what caused it and sent her to an otolaryngologist, who also had no answer. She was referred in recent years to a psychiatrist, a cardiologist and a gastroenterologist. When she was at her regular visit with the psychiatrist, he could not think of a cause. I called her about 5 p.m. one day and we talked for 20 minutes. My first thought was maybe a drug reaction. I wrote down her many medications. Most were drugs I knew but not the two prescribed by the psychiatrist. Looking up the side effects, I found that one of them rarely caused loss of taste. I called the head of the pharmacy at the hospital where I had worked, and though he was unaware of effects, he connected me with the pharmacist who specialized in psychiatric drugs. She immediately told me that the side effect was not common but certainly one they saw more than a few times each year. By now it was almost 6 p.m. when I called Mrs. Bennett back – just 60 minutes. Of course, had I been regularly practicing medicine still and more up-to-date, it would have taken less time. No doctor in a regular practice could have allotted that much time. Yet the answer was right there. She talked to the psychiatrist, and he stopped the medicine. No surprise, her taste came back. Where was her PCP? He was busy seeing many patients each day and did not have the time.

Medicare Readmission Rates as a Marker of Poor Care Coordination

Among individuals on Medicare who are admitted to the hospital, about 20 percent will have an unplanned readmission within 30 days of discharge, with the percentage higher for some conditions such as heart failure. This is an outrageous number and a clear marker of a quality lapse. Why does it happen? There are myriad reasons. Of course, some individuals are severely ill and need readmission no matter the quality of care. But most others are readmitted due to a breakdown in the care delivery system and management of one or more of their chronic illnesses. Perhaps the hospitalist who cared for the patient did not communicate with the primary care doctor upon discharge. Perhaps the instructions to the patient at discharge were complicated and confusing, and the patient did not follow the outlined plan. Perhaps the patient needed a friend or family member to assist with follow-up instructions, to receive and understand those instructions or ask questions of clarification. For some patients, the number of prescription medications is large, which makes an error more likely and compliance difficult at best.

But most important is the lack of good communication between patient and provider. All too often, the PCP does not know his or her patient was in the hospital, learning only when the patient reports it at the next office visit. This is an unacceptable lack of provider-to-provider communication. What is clear is that readmissions are lower if the PCP is actively involved in the discharge, either by being fully up-to-date on the patient's progress and issues during the day of discharge, and maintains continual care of the patient. The possibility of readmission drops dramatically when the patient is seen by his or her primary care physician within a few days after discharge to review medications and review other post hospital plans and other instructions. For example, the Charlestown Erickson Living continuing care retirement community in Maryland schedules a PCP visit within the two-day window after discharge. The readmission rate has fallen and consistently remained under 11 percent in recent years. This reduces the total costs of care dramatically, and when the PCP is intimately involved in coordinating the patient's care, the quality goes up substantially.

In summary, chronic illnesses are commonplace today, and the number of individuals with them is increasing rapidly each year. Diseases such as heart failure, chronic lung or kidney disease and diabetes with complications will last for the rest of the patient's life and need a great deal of attention for excellent care. PCPs are quite competent and experienced to handle most of these diseases most of the time, but they must have time to do so at peak levels. When the time comes for a referral to a specialist, the PCP needs to coordinate that referral. If the patient is admitted to the hospital, there needs to be close consultation between the PCP and the hospitalist throughout the admission, especially at the time of discharge. Patients need to be instructed to visit their PCP within 48 hours of discharge. It is simply not sufficient to tell the patient to see the PCP "soon or if there is a problem." The hospitalist should, but rarely does, accept responsibility for making that appointment before releasing the patient to go home. These steps are critical for high quality care of today's most common medical illnesses.

A well-functioning primary care system means better quality, greater satisfaction and lower total costs. And it means a transition from episodic medical care to true healthcare. If functioning at peak performance it means a further transition to population healthcare.

PART IV
THE TRANSFORMATION OF PRIMARY CARE THROUGH INNOVATION

Primary care needs to transform in order to be the basis of the care delivery system that it should be, to offer the best possible care to the greatest number of people, to allow true healing to occur, and to gain control over the ever rising total costs of health care.

As I have discussed throughout this book, if we want a healthcare system that works, primary care needs to change dramatically and offer the PCP time to spend directly with patients. Part IV will explain how insurance works today, then how primary care physicians themselves and some organizations and businesses – insurance providers, government agencies, employers and retail stores – are transforming primary care in innovative ways, many of which result in a reduced patient load, more time per visit, better patient care, and lower total costs.

Chapter Thirteen

PUTTING HEALTHCARE DECISIONS BACK WHERE THEY BELONG — IN THE HANDS OF YOU AND YOUR DOCTOR

The fundamental change needed to make you the customer of the doctor is to reorder the payment system, taking it back to true insurance. Primary care is generally not expensive and, until the past few decades, it was paid for out of pocket. Heretical perhaps, but it would be useful to go back again to paying the PCP directly.

If we ever hope to improve care and reduce costs, the current insurance model needs to change. Only when we are directly responsible for paying for our own primary healthcare will we be truly accountable. Don't get me wrong. This does not mean no insurance, but rather rethinking what its real benefit should be. Insurance by its name means coverage for the unexpected and expensive, not the routine. It may feel counter-intuitive, but paying your PCP directly and out of pocket — ideally with a tax-advantaged HSA account — will put you, not your insurance company, in true control of your healthcare. And your health will probably benefit as well.

A "County Doctor" explains the problem well:

"I can freeze a couple of warts in less than a minute and send a bill to a patient's commercial insurance for much more money than for a fifteen minute visit to change their blood pressure medication.

"I can chat briefly with a patient who comes in for a dressing change done by my nurse, quickly make sure the wound and the dressing look okay and charge for an office visit. But I cannot bill anything for spending a half hour on the phone with a distraught patient who just developed terrible side effects from his new medication and whose X-ray results suggest he needs more testing.

"Health insurance is not like anything else we call insurance; all other insurance products cover the unexpected and not the expected. Most people never collect on their homeowners' insurance, and most people never total their car. Health insurance, on the other hand, is expected by many to be like a bumper-to-bumper warranty that insulates us from every misfortune or inconvenience by covering everything from the smallest and most mundane to the most catastrophic or esoteric.

"What would it look like if Johnny or Fido puts mud prints on the living room wallpaper and Dad makes a claim on his homeowner's policy? Or if Sally spills chocolate ice cream on the beige upholstery of Mommy's new car and the auto insurance has to pay to have the seats recovered?

"In today's healthcare, everything is potentially a covered service, and there are no incentives to limit one's claims against the insurance companies. I believe we need to make patients view healthcare spending as their business, and the money as their money."[59]

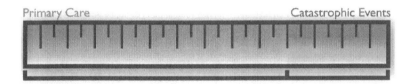

Think of healthcare as a one-foot ruler.[§] About 75 percent, or the first nine inches, represents primary care – routine care that could include complex chronic illnesses, unexpected acute issues and the common and anticipated needs of most of us. The other 25 percent, or the last three inches, represents the unexpected serious problems – what we might call "major medical" and, in a minority of cases, the catastrophic. Today, insurance purports to pay for all of this when in reality insurance should be for the major medical and the catastrophic. That is the whole point of insurance – to deal with the unexpected, highly expensive events in life such as a car crash or house fire. Since today's health insurance covers essentially everything, it is expensive. A major medical/catastrophic policy, on the other hand, is much less expensive. Further, the 75 percent of healthcare considered as primary care does

---

§ I found this ruler analogy on the web site of MedLion (a company that offers direct primary care and discussed in Chapter 16) at www.medlion.com.

not need to cost much. It could cost much less if the system is turned around so the PCP is paid to deliver high quality in a caring, relationship-based model. Said somewhat differently, it is time to stop tinkering around the edges of the current payment system and rethink what primary care should be, how it is delivered and how to pay for it.

In this chapter we will consider the workings of fee-for-service, with all of its currently perceived inequities, capitation, bundled payments, value-based reimbursement, traditional Medicare and Medicare Advantage. Each has its advantages, disadvantages, adherents and detractors.

When we are responsible for our medical payments in some form, we ask more questions ("I don't really understand this diagnosis"), challenge recommendations ("Do I really need that MRI?"), are more willing to try lifestyle modifications rather than insist on a prescription (such as simple measures to prevent heartburn rather than cover it up with Prilosec) and are more accountable. This can be a simple change, such as an employer prefilling an HSA account and then expecting the employee to use the dollars to pay for primary care. The money came from the employer, but now the employees treat it like their own money.

At the same time, price transparency is essential, which is rarely the case today. When you know three different centers charge different amounts for a knee replacement yet have the same outcomes, you can purchase selectively.

It is often stated that if we had a universal payer system the problems would be resolved. But that is not true. Medicare is a universal system for those older than 65, and it has caused most of the problems with primary care and the rising costs of care that are bankrupting the nation. Both political parties know what the problem is, but they cannot find a resolution in this divided time. The Veterans Administration is a universal payer, and recent reports show that has been a disaster. Medicaid is the same. A major problem with each is that they offer essentially unlimited care without patient engagement. Until each person has a sense that it is his or her money, the universal payer concept will not work.

Insurance Should Be Insurance – Not Prepaid Medical Care

The insurance system for healthcare is perverse. But do the insurance companies deserve the blame that is often placed on them for our current state of affairs?

How did we get here? Going back about 100 years, there was limited call for health insurance. Medical care was relatively inexpensive, hospitalizations were uncommon, and it was expected that the individual was responsible. Life insurance and disability insurance were considered more valuable and important in the rapidly-developing industrial world. Then wage and price controls came into effect during World War II, which led unions to push for non-wage benefits such as health insurance. Business reciprocated to be more competitive in the job market without raising salary or wages. The idea was to insure someone for the unexpected, high-cost health event such as major surgery or hospitalization, and the individual still paid for routine care, vaccination, family doctor visits and medications. At that time, patients were still the customer of the physician, especially the primary care physician.

Following World War II, not-for-profit Blue Cross plans for hospitalization insurance and Blue Shield plans for physician coverage developed across the country. But in both cases, the emphasis was on the unexpected, expensive care, not the routine. You (or your parent and grandparents) still paid for everyday care needs and looked to insurance for surgery or hospitalization. But over time employers (including government employers) began to expand coverage to include visits previously paid by the individual, often at the urging of unions and legislators. Concurrently, state legislatures established insurance mandates, which were requirements that had to be covered by any policy sold in that state. Slowly but surely, insurance morphed from "insurance" to prepaid medical care. Of course, premiums increased to pay for the added benefits. As long as your employer (whether business or government) covered the increases in premiums, these were added benefits to you at no extra cost. But that began to erode as companies realized they could no longer afford the premium hikes and asked their employees to cover part of the cost.

Over time, larger companies found it was advantageous to self-insure, especially if their workforce was younger and healthier. They contracted with the insurance company to serve as their third party administrator (TPA) or payer (TPP) for their employees' health care costs and purchased a level of insurance above that for highly unusual and catastrophic events.

As healthcare costs continued to escalate, companies began to expect the employee to pay a portion of the "insurance." Today, non-unionized public companies expect their staff to pay between 25-35 percent of the premiums, and often more. Slowly but surely, governments and unionized companies are doing the same. Add to this the various co-pays and deductibles, which all partially shift more of the costs onto the individual and presumably encourage the employee to be more cost conscious.

Unfortunately, the result is a system where the individual has little direct financial stake in the doctor visit. Small co-pays are mostly an annoyance, although they do reduce the number of visits to the doctor for some patients. Conversely, the doctor knows that the insurer (or TPA) – not the patient – is the one who decides whether and how much he or she will be paid. The primary care doctor, meanwhile, has seen income stay flat or decline in the face of increasing office costs, leading him or her to reduce time per visit to accommodate more visits per day. The result is less satisfactory care and less satisfaction for the patient and the doctor.

Is the insurer at fault for the messy situation? Not really. As a TPA, they are essentially working for the employer within the guidelines set out by the state insurance commissioner and state legislature. They cannot practice medicine. They do not (usually) own the hospital. They do, however, set the rates that the PCP will receive.

For those who buy their insurance directly rather than through an employer, the reforms in the Affordable Care Act, such as the development of exchanges, will not change the critical issue of the doctor-patient contractual relationship. Medicare likewise eliminates this doctor-patient relationship. This is unfortunate because the relationship is key to better personal care.

The ACA mandates a set of 12 "essential services" that every insurance policy must contain. All seem logical and reasonable, but it essentially has further cemented the concept that healthcare insurance is not just insurance but prepaid medical care.

As one of my PCP interviewees reported, "Insurance is a policy we buy to protect us from an unforeseeable situation. However, we are using insurance to pay for foreseeable care. Every diabetic needs to be seen every three months, and a patient needs a yearly comprehensive wellness evaluation and exam. And most people get sick, 2-3x per year that require a doctor's visit – this is all foreseeable even if the exact timing and issue is not foreseeable. Insurance has just become a method of payment but devalues the care we deliver. So when we charge $150, the insurer pays $59 for the visit. In the insurance model of primary care, it's a very expensive form of payment to accept and is quite complicated with tons of red-tape that leads to so much dissatisfaction. No other business out there would operate like this, but physician practices do, as we are an altruistic profession."

High-Deductible Policies

Another option is to obtain a high-deductible insurance policy. This means the premiums come down and you pay for primary care out of pocket. Primary care is generally not expensive, and you are in a position to expect more from the doctor. After all, you are now paying the bill and doing so directly. But actually you and the doctor are still not really in a direct relationship. The PCP still sends the bill to the insurer who in turn sets the allowable reimbursement, then tells you to pay that amount as part of your deductible. It may be a fair price for the service or not but it is still a business relationship between the doctor and the insurer rather than the doctor and you.

High-deductible plans became more common after a 2003 law allowed those who purchased a high-deductible policy to open a health savings account (HSA), and thereby pay health associated costs with tax-advantaged dollars. By 2013, 17 percent of employers offered high-deductible plans, and the number is expected to top 40 percent in 2014.

According to the Centers for Disease Control and Prevention (CDC), 17 percent of those under 65 who had private health insurance policies in 2007 had high deductible policies and 5 percent had consumer-directed health plans (CDHP), which is a combination of a high-deductible policy and an associated HSA. Another 5 percent had a high-deductible plan alone. By 2012, that increased to 11 with a CDHP percent and 20 with a high-deductible only plan for a total of 31 percent with high-deductible plans with or without an HSA. With employers pushing them and the new Affordable Care Act health exchanges offering them, high-deductible plans, especially employer CDHPs, are ascending rapidly. These will be discussed more fully in Chapter 17.

But you might say your primary care is paid for now with your insurance, minus some co-pays and a deductible. Why would you want to give that up and pay out of pocket? Remember the old rule — there is no free lunch. You already pay for it in your premiums. It is better to pay it directly and have a much lower premium for major medical or catastrophic care, and it will actually be cheaper that way.

The Affordable Care Act mandates that approved preventive care, including screenings, should be offered with no deductibles or co-pays by both commercial and government-sponsored insurance. This was done to encourage individuals to get preventive care but not worry about paying for it. These costs are built into the premiums. Of course, the government's concern was that individuals forgo preventive care unless it appears to be "free." If there is no charge, they hoped more people would get preventive care with consequent savings down the road. But obviously preventive care with no co-pays or deductibles means higher premiums. The care must be paid for by someone. Why not let the individual choose to either pay for preventive care directly with lower premiums or have non-deductible/co-pay preventive care with correspondingly higher premiums? When patients pay directly, they have the opportunity to shop around and let the marketplace set the price. Think of Lasik refractive eye surgery, which is not covered by insurance. The price has come down dramatically over time. The price of other preventive services, such as mammograms and colonoscopies, would as well if the price was transparent and the individual paid directly.

I had a colonoscopy recently and cannot say enough positive about the doctor and the staff. They were friendly, efficient, caring and competent. It might be instructive to consider the numbers. The gastroenterologist billed $964, which Medicare reduced to $327.61. The anesthesiologists billed $975, which was reduced to $150. There was a facility charge of $695, which was reduced to $391. The total charges were $2,634 and Medicare allowed $888.61. I have no idea what the "appropriate" price should be, but I am certain that if everyone paid directly, the price would come down through market forces. Maybe Medicare brought it down to the right price point. Personally, I think it is better to not have a centralized bureaucracy determine the price — let the market drive the process. Left unfettered, it can work well.

There is a strong need now to change the professional relationship so patients have an incentive to take control of their doctor-patient relationships.

Direct payment for primary care services creates the appropriate professional-client relationship that encourages the PCP to deliver quality and service and gives patients the responsibility of taking ownership of their own health and wellness. These are changes in the delivery system that need to occur, and the sooner the better.

There are some important caveats to high-deductible policies. The doctor must still submit a claim form to the insurer so the insurer knows the service was rendered and subtracts that amount from the remaining deductible. The insurer only deducts the amount it would have paid had there been no deductible. For example, the PCP could give extensive time to you and charge appropriately, with your understanding and acceptance. But the doctor may have a contract with the insurer that requires him or her to abide by the insurer's reimbursement rates. This is a conundrum unless the physician decides to not accept any insurance payments, charges you appropriately and gives you a form to send in yourself to the insurer. As a result, the bill to you is $200, but the insurer says a visit is only reimbursed at $100. So you spend $200 but your deductible is only reduced by $100.

In my interviews with PCPs, they had mixed views of high-deductible policies and retainer-based practices. Many said high deductibles are appropriate and generally a good idea. Others were concerned that some patients might be unable to pay for care and avoid a visit. Conversely, some suggested that each patient should choose the level of deductible most appropriate for them – just as one does with auto collision insurance. "Let me buy the level of coverage I need for my current station in life." They noted that most people do not appreciate the current insurance model that pays for the routine, not just the highly expensive or the catastrophic, with the cost of the routine built into the insurance premiums. Of course, if someone else pays the premiums (such as the employer or Medicare Part B and D and Medigap), then it is to the patient's advantage to not have a high deductible. Connecting the high deductible with an HSA, including with Medicare which currently does not allow HSAs, seemed to be a logical approach to many.

The value of high deductibles, according to many of the PCPs, is that it encourages patients to ask more questions and become better informed about their health and treatments. Many believed a market-driven model makes more sense than the current system. They believed that when PCPs have a set and transparent fee schedule and the patient pays directly, the relationship between patient and doctor strengthens.

In my interviews with PCPs, they also said in various ways that there needs to be transparency in pricing. Today they might have a set fee for a visit, but each insurer has its own contract and sets the reimbursement, which results in all different fees. The PCP finds it difficult to explain the various rates when a patient comes in and asks why his total bill was $125 when his neighbor who has a different insurer had a bill of $100 for the same type of visit.

The responses varied about paying the PCP out of pocket, and it was clear that many had not given this substantial thought. On the one hand, PCPs generally thought it was a viable option but were concerned that many patients could not afford to pay out of pocket for primary care. This was a concern especially for patients with chronic illnesses who need to see the physician frequently.

One PCP said he favored a universal payer with everything included, but then he noted that the epitome of a universal payer, Medicare, was often a "nightmare to work with." Others, each in a "regular" primary care practice, referred to the retainer-based concept as a means to provide more time and hence better care. But they were concerned that many individuals could not afford the retainer. Another felt that retainer-based practices were elitist, but "Hey, it a free country." Still others, usually those in membership/retainer practices, pointed to low costs and suggested that the Affordable Care Act effectively encouraged retainer/membership practices under the high-deductible Bronze plans offered in the exchanges. For example, direct primary care (retainer/membership) is "growing to meet the need of the underinsured and uninsured. It is growing to meet the need for highly personalized care, where the doctor remembers the patient's name. And it allows PCPs to get their voices back and to be the masters of their professions."

Fee-For-Service

Fee-for-service is the way medical care has been paid for centuries, basically like any other profession or service provider. The big exception is that in health care the doctor and the recipient are not in charge of the business arrangement. There is at least one intermediary and often more, including the insurer, the employer or the government.

The current fee-for-service model is broken. Many policy experts believe the fee-for-service approach means excessive utilization with increased use of specialist referrals, tests, procedures and hospitalizations. I believe this is correct but for a different reason. The PCP is paid too little per patient visit and is burdened with too many patients to give high quality comprehensive primary care. This rapidly drives up the total costs of care with excess referrals, tests and even hospitalizations.

Here is a patient story that exemplifies this conundrum: Sampson is a highly-regarded professional with a PhD in his field but remarkably minimal medical knowledge. Same for his wife. He had multiple chronic medical conditions, including chronic lung disease, congestive heart failure, moderate kidney failure, diabetes, and hypertension, which meant multiple medications. Remarkably, he was functional most of the time and was able to continuously conduct his professional activities. He had a long-time PCP, but she generally gave him 10-15 minutes of time during each visit, so he only went to her when he had an acute flare-up of one of his chronic diseases. One day he developed an acute exacerbation of his breathing problems, called his PCP and was told to go directly to the emergency room. She did not call the ER physician and give any information about his medical history. Sampson was found to have pneumonia, admitted and cared for by a hospitalist who also had no contact with the PCP. On discharge a week later, he was given prescriptions for seventeen (yes, 17) medications. His wife picked them up at the pharmacy, and he followed the directions. He had not been instructed to make a prompt appointment with his PCP, nor did he think he needed to go back to his PCP unless he had a new problem. He was soon back in the hospital. Why? Although the pneumonia had been well-treated, some of his other problems had gotten out of control. In addition, one prescription had an incorrect dose schedule – three times rather than one time per day. Had he seen his PCP shortly after discharge and had she given him the time needed to review his situation, she would have realized that his multiple other diseases needed attention and resolved the medication error. This might have been rectified in time to prevent another hospitalization.

Doctors invoice insurance carriers for an amount that may be commensurate with the service delivered. But that does not matter because the insurer is the arbiter of the payment, offering an amount that it deems appropriate based on a coding system. This coding system, called CPT and ICD-9 and soon ICD-10, must be followed. For instance, an earache has a specific code number. An earache and a sore throat has another code. This system assumes that it is possible to categorize any type of provider-patient interaction with a specific code number, and the insurer reimburses by code number. This sounds fine but it negates the value of time – time to listen deeply, time to think or time to consult with a peer. A PCP can spend 10 minutes or 30 minutes with you, but it is still an earache and has a fixed code. A physician no longer bills the patient for the time and effort spent. The system pushes for short visits. Cognitive activities are not valued. [For a brief description of the coding system, see the endnote.][60]

Capitation

Various alternatives to fee-for-service have been proposed, most based on a fixed amount per patient per year (capitation), a fixed amount per episode of care (such as a heart attack or gall bladder removal, often called bundling) or converting to a full-salary model for the PCP.

With capitation, the insurer pays the doctor a set amount per month or year for all primary care. This is not inherently different than the retainer-based model (see Chapter 14) except for one key variation – with capitation, the payer is the insurer and with retainer-based care, the payer is the patient. In the latter, the patient is willing to pay because he is promised a practice of about 500-800 patients along with certain practice characteristics – same-day appointments, visits as long as needed, and the PCP's cell phone for after-hours issues. These benefits justify the cost for those who choose it. The insurer capitation model only leads to high quality care if the insurer pays enough per patient (the "cap" rate) to keep the practice at a limit of about 500-1,000 total individuals, the preferable number depending on the health status of the patient population.

PCPs told me that in the days of managed care capitation in the 1990s, since a patient could only access a specialist with the blessing of the PCP, unnecessary direct visits to specialists were initially down. But for many, capitation backfired because the PCP was given too large a group to care for and had too little time for each patient, so the PCP referred the patient to the specialist anyway, driving up costs rather than figuring out the problem. It seems the insurers may still not have learned this lesson. Today, most insurers do not recognize limited patients per primary care doctor as an advantage because they are unconvinced that the total expenditures will decrease.

Bundled Payments

Many healthcare policy leaders believe that "bundling," or aggregating fee-for-service reimbursements, will result in lower total costs. Aggregation can take the form of capitation for a year of care, or it can be tied to an "episode" of care – a total knee replacement, for example, where a fixed amount is made available for the surgery, hospitalization, post-operative rehabilitation, and medications. It is then up to the various involved parties to agree on the distribution of the funds among themselves. Knee and hip replacements for osteoarthritis are good examples because they are discrete episodes and top the list of health expenditures among Medicare enrollees at 5.7 percent of spending, or $7.3 billion per year. Other discrete episodes of care include heart valve replacement, coronary artery bypass surgery, pneumonia, or a fractured hip. But the valve replacement might be for a patient with congestive heart failure that will last for the rest of the patient's life, and the bypass surgery might be part of the overall care of someone with a heart attack. These and other diagnoses are less likely, in my opinion, to work in a bundled fashion. Individuals with chronic illnesses have acute episodes that fall into these categories, but the ongoing care of the patient by the PCP and specialists would not fit this rubric well.

Nevertheless, a study of Medicare payments and diagnoses showed that among 245 diagnostic groupings, 17 (with joint replacements at the top of the list) represented one-half of all payments for care and five accounted for almost 25 percent during a recent year. The costs varied across the country without any apparent relationship to quality outcomes. Further analysis suggested that if the bundled payment was set at the 25th percentile of current total fee-for-service payments for that episode of care, the savings for these top 17 diagnoses would be $10 billion less per year. If the payment was set at the 50th percentile, the savings would be $4.7 billion.[61]

Salaried Models

Many organizations, especially hospitals and some insurance plans, employ physicians on a salaried basis. In fact, hospitals are aggressively seeking PCPs to become employees. An employed PCP means downstream revenue for the hospital. Most physician employers, including hospitals, pay the PCP a salary with certain bonus opportunities. But the hospital must bill insurers on a fee-for-service basis on behalf of the PCP, so they set productivity standards that require the PCP to see too many patients for too short a period of time each. The quality suffers and the patient-doctor relationship is never adequate for either the patient or the doctor. However, the hospital, under today's fee-for-service approach, is pleased because the PCP makes use of its laboratories, radiology services and specialists and admits his or her patients to the hospital. Since hospitals have clout with the insurers, they can often obtain a better reimbursement rate than the PCP is able to do alone in practice. But many insurers have observed that the total costs of care increase when the PCP is employed rather than in a private practice.

Traditional Medicare

Medicare, which is the country's major insurer by total dollars expended, primarily pays via a fee-for-service model. As part of the Affordable Care Act, Medicare's primary care fee-for-service reimbursements will rise over time by about 10 percent. This is not enough to change practice patterns. Doctors will readily accept the cash but not reduce the number of patients under their care nor lengthen the visit times, so there will be no quality improvement, no reduction in referrals to specialists, no reduction in total health care expenditures and no improvement in patient satisfaction. The patient can never become the doctor's customer since Medicare continues to set the rates and decides whether a service is covered or not. Medicare does not have high-deductible policies and does not allow enrollees to have health savings accounts. If Medicare's cost structures are not remodeled, it will ultimately bankrupt the country. More importantly, Americans will not obtain the care they deserve or thought they would get after years of paying into the Medicare Trust Fund.

Medicare has recently announced with substantial fanfare that it will, over the next few years, migrate from the current fee for service model to a fee for quality or fee for outcomes approach.[62] While this "value-based" payment concept is laudable, many physicians are highly skeptical. Medicare sets out numerous bureaucratic hurdles that currently drive up the PCPs' cost of practice and deprive the doctor of time spent with the patient. Their concern is that new models will only exacerbate this problem. Here are just a few of the issues PCPs (and other doctors) deal with daily.

The electronic medical record is an important tool but its implementation has been nothing but frustrating to most PCPs. Medicare requires that a doctor must be in substantial compliance with its "meaningful use" requirements or else the doctor will get reduced reimbursements. Sounds appropriate until you learn that many PCPs say it takes them an extra hour per day to get their charts in order to be compliant. Another effort that is not direct patient care.

Medicare has quality indicators that must be met. There are standard, well accepted quality measures such as levels of Hemoglobin A1c (a measure of diabetes care) or blood pressure control. Quality measures sound appropriate but are they really the ones that matter the most to actual older patients? Or just more paperwork added to an already overburdened PCP?

Patients are clear that what *they* most care about are quality time with their physician, time to develop a relationship, time to be listened to and to build trust. They want easy access with short waits, a cheerful receptionist and a sense that they are the true customer of the doctor. That is of course impossible if the doctor has only fifteen minutes per patient.

The HA1c or blood pressure measurements may be low resulting in a plus mark with Medicare. But if the patient wakes up with a blood glucose of 70 and feels groggy that's hardly quality. If the blood pressure is low it counts as a plus but if the patient has resultant syncope, falls, breaks a hip and is hospitalized, that does not count as bad quality. Something is perverse here.[63]

A related problem is the coming use of ICD-10 coding. Currently there are about 18,000 discrete codes – for example, anemia is coded 280 and anemia from Plummer-Vincent Syndrome is 280.8. That system is bad enough. With ICD-10 the number of codes will rise to about 140,000. A dog bite, for example, is coded W540XXA and a cat bite is W5501XA. A bite by a parrot is W6101XA but if it was a macaw bite the code is W6111XA. And so on; bureaucracy run totally amuck. Imagine the time that will need to be spent looking up the proper code for each problem. Want to bet that more and more physicians will choose not to participate in Medicare? Will this be the added straw that finally breaks the camel's back?

Medicare is not free nor is it complete in its coverage. Part A (mostly hospital care) is covered by the Medicare Trust Fund through the Medicare tax on income that you paid throughout your working lifetime. The 2.9 percent of earned income is divided equally between you and your employer or is fully paid by you if self-employed. There is no additional premium expense to the individual once on Medicare's rolls but there are deductibles and co-pays. Part B (mostly physicians' care and other out-patient care) is paid 50-50 percent by the federal government and the individual. For most people it costs about $103 per month subtracted from your Social Security payments. The premiums are greater for those with higher incomes. Part D drug coverage benefits are also jointly paid by the government, with the individual paying about $37 per month as of 2014. This can vary from as low as $12 per month with high deductibles and high co-pays to more than $100 per month with lower deductibles but still significant co-pays. A Medigap policy for the 25 percent of services that Medicare A and B do not cover costs about $225-300 per month as well. There are multiple plan levels with lower premiums resulting in lower payments, but premiums increase with advancing age. A retired couple will spend a minimum of $6,000 – probably more like $10,000 – annually for their combined Medicare/Medigap/drug coverage, plus deductibles, co-pays and, importantly, non-covered services such as routine vision, hearing and dental care. A Medigap policy does not assist with these non-covered services, only the portion of services that Medicare considers covered services but does not reimburse.

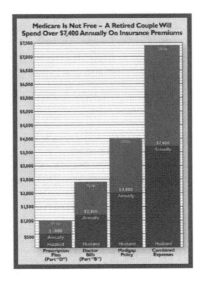

Dr. Andy Lazris, a geriatrician, told me this story about a patient (which he also describes in his book *Curing Medicare*.) She was 98 years old, somewhat demented but happy in her assisted living community. One night she was noted to be weak and confused. The nurses sent her to the emergency room where she had multiple blood tests run and a CT scan of the head. She became more confused in the hospital and had to be sedated. Eventually she was found to have a urinary tract infection, was treated and sent back. Medicare paid for her ER visit, the testing, the CT scan. Dr. Lazris noted that she could have been kept at the assisted living facility, not been subjected to multiple testing which only further confused and frightened her. But having a doctor on call to see her late at night would be expensive and the costs would not be fully recouped from Medicare. It was more cost effective to send her to the ER where Medicare would pick up the bill. Further, our medical care system has a tendency to push for aggressive diagnosis and treatment as was done with the blood tests and CT scan even when it is probably not to the person's benefit. Again, Medicare will pay for all those tests and the ER visit even though a cheaper and more humane approach would have worked and been more appropriate. Although she was not admitted to the hospital, a person in her circumstances often is and then, because of the way Medicare works, sent to a nursing home. There Medicare will pay for 100 days of care provided she was in the hospital for at least three days. Medicare will not pay to care for her if she is returned to the assisted living facility even though that might be a more effective and appropriate approach. The point here is that Medicare actually encourages high cost medical care, a type of medical care that is not necessarily in the best interest of the older patient.[27]

Medicare Advantage

Medicare Advantage uses both fee-for-service and capitation as payment models. Currently, about one-quarter of Medicare enrollees join a Medicare Advantage (Part C) plan operated by private insurers. These plans combine Part A, Part B, Medigap, a prescription drug plan and other services (vision, hearing, dental) at a price considerably below the minimum $6,000 a year in premiums for a retired couple. The individual still pays the Part B premium, which is taken directly out of Social Security payments each month.

Some Medicare Advantage plans pay a fee-for-service reimbursement to the physician, and some use a capitated approach to pay the primary care physician a flat rate per year. A few pay a "cap rate" high enough that the PCP can afford to reduce his or her practice size to a more manageable number. We will look at this in some detail in a later chapter.

It is likely, perhaps inevitable, that the number of Medicare enrollees in Medicare Advantage plans will increase with time. Enrollees today are largely those with their retirement needs covered by defined contribution 401(k)s, IRAs and personal savings. Many enrollees are those who worked in the service industry and have little in the way of retirement funding. Medicare Advantage saves them substantial money or gives more coverage compared to Traditional Medicare. Traditional (or regular) Medicare enrollees almost always include individuals who have government, large corporate or union-negotiated pensions because their Part B, Medigap and Part D Drug benefits are paid as part of their retirement benefits. This is a savings of $6,000 or more per year for a retired couple. Those with typical pensions find no further advantage with Part C plans. But many companies are dropping their health benefits for retirees and sending them to the new exchanges; they may prefer Medicare Advantage if only for the cost savings. As more individuals retire with defined contribution retirement funds, which have no built-in health benefits, they will likely gravitate to Medicare Advantage (Part C) plans rather than Traditional Medicare. This will drive up the percentage and absolute numbers on Advantage plans, thus pushing down the percentage on Traditional Medicare.

In my view, insurance should be insurance, not prepaid medical care. But that is not what has transpired over the years in American healthcare insurance. When insurance pays for all healthcare rather than unexpected "major medical" and catastrophic illnesses, it eliminates market forces and places the burden of cost management on the insurers. They, in turn, have responded with price controls. It has not worked and has marginalized the ability of PCPs to offer expanded comprehensive primary care with consequent wellness and health preservation. Medical care costs continue to rise and so do healthcare insurance costs. Putting patients – and their PCPs – in charge will change that.

CHAPTER FOURTEEN

INNOVATORS: PRIMARY CARE PHYSICIANS WHO GOT IT RIGHT

Primary care today is a production-line approach akin to the famous *I Love Lucy* segment where Lucy and Ethyl are wrapping chocolates on a conveyor line: they wrapped as fast as they could and pretended to keep up, even though they could not.[64]

With a fast-moving conveyor, the job cannot be done properly. Slowing down the conveyor leads to better quality. It may cost more to get the job done, but there are fewer chocolates improperly wrapped or falling on the floor, so the total costs go down.

As I have stated, the fundamental problem in primary care delivery today is not enough time for each patient. There is a highly dysfunctional payment system that leads to higher costs, less quality and reduced satisfaction. The core problem? Too many patients per day per doctor, secondary to price controls and regulations that have reduced the time, trust and core interactions between doctor and patient. The patient is no one's customer and visit times are too short.

Some of the best attempts to improve this dysfunctional delivery system have been accomplished by primary care physicians who have fundamentally said they "won't take it any longer" and have opted for a new, better system rather than wait for others to fix it for them. They have been the innovators and have changed the paradigm so they can offer each patient as much time as necessary – no more rushed visits for the patient and no more long days of 25 patients per PCP. Here are some of those innovations.

Direct Primary Care

The concept of direct primary care is to remove the insurer as the payer for primary care and replace it with a payment model that allows patients to pay PCPs directly and PCPs to reduce their number of patients to 500-800, sometimes even less if the patients are mostly severely ill. With fewer patients, each gets longer visit times, easy access and comprehensive primary care.

Direct primary care takes many forms, and there are two principle payment systems. In one, the patient pays the doctor for each visit, usually at a rate far below the insurance model because the doctor now has dramatically reduced overhead costs. This is sometimes called *direct pay* or "pay at the door," not unlike the way it was until a few decades ago. Under the second model, the patient purchases a package of care paid monthly or annually. This basic model comes with many variations and is called *direct primary care, membership, retainer-based* or *concierge medicine*. They all have certain characteristics in common but vary in how the practice functions. Some argue that each is inherently different, but they are actually quite similar, especially in offering the patient more time. Although direct primary care (DPC) implies renouncing insurance, many DPC practices actually still accept insurance. Concierge Medicine Today estimates that about 8,000 direct primary care physicians practice in the U.S.[65] About 1 percent of PCPs are switching to some form of direct pay practice annually, and the number is growing rapidly.[66] If the PCP has a reduced patient size, he or she can offer same or next-day appointments that last as long as necessary, email communication, and 24/7 cell phone availability. Most offer unlimited same-day or next-day office visits, no copays and no added charges for minor procedures (such as laceration stitching or removal of a mole). Some make house calls and nursing home visits for no extra charge, and others add a modest cash fee.

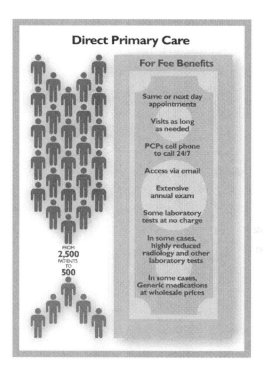

Direct Primary Care

For Fee Benefits

Same or next day appointments

Visits as long as needed

PCPs cell phone to call 24/7

Access via email

Extensive annual exam

Some laboratory tests at no charge

In some cases, highly reduced radiology and other laboratory tests

In some cases, Generic medications at wholesale prices

FROM **2,500** PATIENTS TO **500**

In any of these practices, an arrangement may allow patients to obtain laboratory testing, imaging and procedures at highly discounted rates from selected vendors. Some practices offer a limited number of laboratory tests at no charge, and others supply generic medications at no or wholesale cost. For the patient with multiple prescription medications, the savings on drug costs can more than offset the annual subscription expense of direct primary care.

These practices tend to be quite selective when they refer to specialists. They tend to work with like-minded specialists who offer extended visit times and highly discounted, transparent fees for those who pay cash, have high-deductible plans or have no insurance at all.

Often regarded as being only for the "1 percent," direct primary care practices can be affordable and a good choice for those with no insurance, limited insurance, or modest incomes. Consider it "blue collar" concierge medicine.

With a direct primary care arrangement with the physician, patients can buy a high-deductible "catastrophic" policy with much lower premiums for unexpected expensive needs. I have argued in the *Washington Times* Op-Ed section that paying the doctor directly is better for all concerned.[67] Patients take a more active role in the entire care process, and the doctor allots meaningful time for patient interaction. This is a return to "relationship medicine."

According to a 2014 Kaiser Family Foundation report, about 31 percent of employers now offer high-deductible health plans with a HSA so routine care can be paid with tax-advantaged dollars. About 20 percent of employer-covered workers signed up for such plans in 2013 and the trend is continuing upward.[68] The new health exchanges created by the Affordable Care Act also have high deductible plans available, which in turn allow for creation of an HSA and use of tax-advantaged dollars for health care expenses, although premium payments probably cannot be paid thorough the HSA. Dollars placed in an HSA and not used in one year can be rolled forward to subsequent years so no money is lost.

When your money is used, you command more physician time – valuable time needed to do careful assessments, call a specialist, describe the rationale for the referral, and request a prompt appointment with that specialist. When you pay directly, you get more of the doctor's time and expertise. You also engage with the doctor: "Do I really need to take that test, visit that specialist or take that prescription?" "Will the result of that test alter my care?" "Are you just doing this as defensive medicine?" Questions like these lead to better care and lower costs, and defensive medicine likely declines substantially. With your own money at stake, there is an incentive to get cost effective care. In this model, your doctor appreciates that it is your money and will try to keep your costs as low as possible. You are now the doctor's client, the insurer is no longer the customer.

Dr. Steven Horvitz, a direct primary care practice physician in Moorestown, NJ, sent me this comment: "I find in my practice it is the time spent with my patients that allows for less defensive medicine. More time, more explanations, more questions asked and answered, gets closer to a true working diagnosis and treatment. Doctors of yesteryear were probably more skilled than today as they did NOT utilize as many tests for diagnosis.

They used common sense, skill and longer patient interactions. So maybe the money buys more physician time, but it is really the time that allows for less defensive medicine."

A PCP in a typical insurance-based practice spends over 50% percent of collections on administrative costs for coding, billing and collections, dollars not spent on direct care of the patient.[69] Given today's insurance reimbursement rates, the physician nets about $27 to $34 per visit after expenses and must see 20-30 patients per day to cover overhead and still maintain income. This suggests that a large amount of money could be saved by eliminating the administrative costs and contracting directly with the patient as a customer.

Direct Pay Practices

Direct pay practices (sometimes called "cash only") are essentially a return to the past, which expects the patient to pay a fee for each visit – "pay at the door." Doctors who use this model charge a reduced amount because they no longer have the substantial costs of billing and collections yet still earn a good income while reducing the number of patients to a more manageable number.

Some doctors now post a price list on the Internet for all to see. This creates transparency and gives patients the dignity of knowing in advance what the cost of a visit may be. For example, one direct pay physician posts that a drained abscess is $30, a Pap smear is $40, ingrown toenail removal is $50, and a 30-minute house call is $100. Since he has no staff for coding and billing the insurer and accepts only a credit card, cash or check, his costs are lower and he can afford to offer reasonable prices. This same physician allows his patients to consult with him via email or Skype for a monthly fee of $20-30. Some might compare this to airlines charging extra for a checked bag or an onboard snack, but the idea is to promote a direct, clear understanding of the costs upfront at a price that is considerably less than through insurance. For example, if you have a high-deductible policy and see your PCP in a regular practice, the bill to the insurer is usually higher than if your PCP does not participate in insurance and bills you directly. In these practices, the doctor can give you a form that spells out the services so you can submit it to the insurance company for payment or credit toward the deductible. Of course, this represents a new hassle for you and can lead to reduced patient satisfaction.

Here is how one physician, Dr. Michael Henderson of Oregon, described direct primary care. "DPC is about restoring a healthy *patient-doctor relationship* (emphasis mine). It is about physicians being able to provide patients the healthcare services they need — not inappropriate care, under care or overutilization the current system promotes. It is about getting rid of the [misaligned incentives] of the insurance industry. It is about making insurance actually function like insurance, not prepaid medical services/insurance. What the numbers don't show is why there are so many referrals [from PCPs to specialists.] Anything that takes slightly more time is referred to a specialist to keep the PCP's volume up. PCPs are practicing production-line medicine and are not practicing to the full extent of our training. The current insurance model rewards mediocre, expensive care – not providing effective, coordinated care that patients need. Patients need time, which is very difficult to provide… DPC allows me to work for the patient and do what I am trained to do. That is why I went into medicine."[70]

Membership, Retainer and Concierge Models of Direct Primary Care

Many PCPs prefer to have the convenience of a monthly or annual payment rather than collect after each visit. Membership, retainer or concierge models seek that difference. The terms "direct primary care" and "membership" are traditionally divided from "retainer" and "concierge" based on total cost and whether fees are paid monthly or annually. The practices work the same way but vary in the services provided. With these caveats, here is a discussion of direct/membership plans, followed by retainer/concierge plans.

Direct Primary Care/Membership

Fees vary by practice, area of the country, local demographics and age (as a proxy for chronic illnesses) but tend to range from $50-100 per month, even less for children. Sometimes there is a small added payment per visit in practices with the lowest monthly fees. At this rate, the PCP can reduce the patient panel size to 500-800 and still maintain an income equivalent to a 2,500-patient practice size in the old model. When you join a membership practice and combine it with a high-deductible insurance policy and an HSA, the end result can be lower costs for you yet better care. Here are a few examples.

In eastern North Carolina, Atlantic Integrated Health (AIH) has a $50 monthly fee and a $15 charge per visit with an emphasis on health and wellness.[71]

Patient Care Direct (PCD), based in North Carolina, requires patients to pay a monthly membership fee to purchase an "access card." PCD thinks of this like a gym membership with a monthly fee. The office now only needs the clinical team and a receptionist. The doctor does not overtly reduce his or her patient numbers, but patients expect a high level of service that leads to an "appropriate" patient number, according to their spokesperson. Since the practice no longer employs two or three people for billing functions, those dollars can go toward better care delivery, more extensive prevention management and closely coordinating chronic illness care, the spokesperson told me. PCD has developed a wraparound policy called Employer Health Ownership Plan that employers can purchase which offers personalized direct primary care with no added co-pays plus moderate deductible insurance for specialty and hospital care. They argue that this is less expensive than typical insurance, saving the employer and the employee/patients substantially while offering superior care.

Doctors at Atlas MD in Wichita, Kansas, think of themselves as "blue collar" concierge practices. "We realized that insurance paying for primary care is akin to using car insurance to try to pay for gasoline," says Dr. Doug Nunamaker, Atlas MD's chief medical officer. "It's something that's otherwise fairly affordable until you try to pay for it with insurance: My premiums would be much higher because they wouldn't know how much gas I would need, they would tell me where to get gas, and I'd have to preauthorize trips out of town." At Atlas MD, physicians have only 600 patients each under care. Members who are 20-44 years old pay $50 a month, 45-64 pay $75 a month, and 65 and older pay $100 a month. Children and teens up to 19 years old pay $10 a month. A typical family of four, in short, pays about

$120 a month, or $1,440 per year. The membership covers most elements of primary care, from physicals and EKGs to strep tests and stitches. The doctors even do house calls at no extra charge. Medicine and lab work carry wholesale prices: $5 for heartburn medication, for example, or $6 for a prescription to treat migraines. Blood work that might cost $30 out of pocket under an insurance plan instead costs just $2. "I can order-in medicines because the clinic's income is based on membership," Nunamaker explains. "I don't need to make money dispensing medications — I can get 1,000 [generic] Prilosec pills for $55, and I can dispense them to you for a couple dollars. It's significantly less expensive."[72]

In Erie, a working class city in northwestern Pennsylvania, the Izbicki brothers, Jon and Harry, began such as "blue collar" membership practice. Just out of training in family medicine in 2005, they first worked for a health center and later the local hospital. They found that they lost all autonomy and were frequently scolded for not using enough of the hospital's ancillary services – laboratory, imaging and more. So they started their own practice using the typical insurance-based business model. They soon had slightly more than 3,500 patients between them. About 10 percent were Medicare enrollees, which created about 20 percent of the office visits, 50 percent of the hospital visits and perhaps 90 percent of the total work effort. Once again, they were back to seeing too many patients for too short a time. They worked a full day but then spent hours after closing to complete paperwork. Their overhead expenses amounted to about 70 percent of total expenses. "We found that the insurance-based model of primary care is unsustainable. In a price-fixed situation like in health care, the only way to increase your income is to produce more volume, number of units seen per day, a.k.a. the cattle drive."

"We were bitter, frustrated and in eminent danger of become indifferent physicians. We were in a failed profession. It was so bad that we really had to take a risk," says Jon Izbicki, DO.[73] "We knew that what patients want more than anything else is uninterrupted time with their PCP and with that to build a level of confidence in their care. They want relationship-centered care."

After talking with the doctors at AtlasMD and others, with some trepidation, they announced their transition to direct primary care in June 2013 and converted in September 2013. They chose to call their practice "direct primary care" rather than "membership" or "retainer-based" given the fiscal conservatism of Erie. Not all of their patients were pleased, and most did not join the new practice. About 500, or 15 percent, transferred, 2,000 declined and 1,000 did not respond. Many thought it meant paying twice for medical care – once for the insurance and then once more for the PCP. "We took the negative comments and tried to respond positively. We showed that we could bring value, especially with the wholesale medication prices." Over the course of the next 12 months, their practice numbers climbed to about 760 patients between them. They would like to build up to about 600 each.

The Izbicki brothers charge $780 per year, payable as $65 monthly or annually with a discount. They point out that this is about $2 per day for unlimited primary care. This includes everything: wellness care, episodic needs, stitches. Visits are as long as needed and usually the same or next day.

Since they do not contract with any insurers, they have been able to develop contracts with a clinical laboratory and a local imaging center for highly discounted testing and radiology. "The national laboratory we use knows we pay within a week of their monthly invoice. It brings their overheads way down, so they contract with us to afford our DPC office a very cost-effective solution for lab testing for our patients. We collect for the lab testing at the time from our patients so we have no cash flow issues. The result is a bill that might have been $500 is now just $20 to $30. We see this as a value-added service that often can save our patients the cost of their annual membership fee. It can be financially valuable, particularly to the increasing number of individuals with high-deductible policies."

They also have the ability to purchase generic drugs at wholesale prices and sell them to their patients at the same price. For many patients, especially those with multiple chronic illnesses who are taking 5-7 prescription medications, this can save as much as the annual membership fee. This factor encourages Medicare enrollees to join. Dr. Jon Izbicki notes that many older patients on limited fixed incomes cannot afford their prescriptions, even with a Medicare Part D policy, and ration them out by not taking them as prescribed. This often means a medical problem develops, such as exacerbation of heart failure or chronic lung disease, and then "they end up in the ER and admitted into the hospital. We can usually save them substantial amounts of money and make it truly affordable to be compliant and remain healthier as a result. So our price may be $65 but the actual cost per month is way less. This is obviously better health care but it is also saving the entire healthcare system in *total costs* of care.

"In the old system, if I saw an elderly patient with multiple issues and spent 30 minutes with her, I would get $70 from the insurer. If my next patient needed a cerumen [ear wax] extraction, I would get paid $54 yet only spend a few minutes. What a system!

"Today, I am prepaid and I can spend whatever time is necessary with each patient. In the past, if I used liquid nitrogen to remove actinic keratoses [to prevent later possible skin cancer] from the scalp, I would bill $120 for the first lesion and $20 for each additional one. A simple laceration that took five minutes to sew up was paid as $140 and a suture removal was $40. And the patient who had a high-deductible insurance policy would get billed these amounts. There were lots of these examples where the patient got an added expense despite their insurance. So they end up paying twice anyway, for their insurance and for the out-of-pocket that was not covered or applied to deductible. Now it is at no extra charge.

"By the way, we are not primary care physicians but actually complex care physicians. Most people do not realize the extent and breadth of our training and expertise and how little we actually need to refer to specialists when we have the time to take care of it ourselves. Perhaps the term 'complex care physician' would be better than 'primary care physician,' as it more closely relates the work of the doctor, especially with these patients with highly complex, serious illnesses."

Like others who have converted to direct primary care, they are beginning to see employers choosing to either pay the annual retainer for their employees or moving into high-deductible health insurance plans coupled with an HSA to purchase the membership. Dr. Izbicki notes that pairing a high-deductible policy with its much lower premium and a membership with their practice can save as much as 60 percent from a typical insurance policy with a lower deductible.

Not everyone has a sizable practice from which to convert. Most PCPs in practice today are trying to find an "out" from the frustrations of the current system. Since they likely already have a large practice of 2,500 or more patients, switching to the membership or retainer practice makes sense. For younger physicians, however, with no base of patients to draw from, it can be a challenge to get started.

In Lawrence, Kansas, Dr. Ryan Neuhofel began a membership practice right out of his residency training in 2012.[74] He decided while in medical school and residency that he did not want to be in a typical insurance-based practice. "I saw that most physicians did not have fulfilling careers. I saw that they spent enormous time in administrative tasks rather than actually working with their patients. I knew I wanted to do primary care, but it had to be in a model that let me earn a decent living yet let me give really quality care in a compassionate manner. It was a real gamble to go straight into this.

"It's hard to build this type of practice. I had no patients and no reputation in Lawrence. It was not my hometown. So I gave talks at local organizations. I sat on street corners with a humorous sign, anything to get the word out. I moonlighted at a nearby hospital to make ends meet. My practice built slowly at first but is gaining momentum now."[75]

The demographics of his locale are folks with less than the national median income, so his practice is "more like a safety net clinic." About 70-80 percent are uninsured and a large number have complex, chronic illnesses – "a lot more than I anticipated." His monthly fee is $30-40, depending on age, with $100 for a family of four and $10 for each additional child. There are no additional fees except for an after-hours visit or a home visit. Like some other direct primary care practices, he buys medications in bulk from wholesalers and resells to his patients for what he pays plus a small markup for administration. As with the Izbicki brothers, he finds that the savings for some of his patients with multiple prescriptions can be literally hundreds of dollars per month for a family, far outweighing the monthly membership fee. A few employers have noticed and decided to offer his services as a benefit to their employees who take out a high-deductible policy. "I prefer to have a direct financial relationship with my patients, but most employed folks prefer to have their employer take care of the membership payment. I see it as a real source of growth for my practice and the real long-term growth for the whole direct primary care concept. It allows employers to initiate a high-deductible policy yet give the employee access to quality primary care at no added cost. This is especially important for the person with lots of chronic illnesses personally or in the family."

Asked if he was charging enough to make ends meet once his practice grew to its projected size, he said that he may have to increase his prices somewhat but not by much if his practice tops out at 800 patients. But if it grows to a maximum of 1,000, which he is not sure he wants to do, then he will be satisfied with his current pricing structure. "I will be earning about average for a family practice physician in this area and that is just fine with me."

Retainer-Based ("Concierge") Practices

Another direct primary care approach is the retainer-based model, which is sometimes known as concierge medicine. It is essentially the same as the membership model but with a different name and perhaps a few more services. As with the other plans, the physician no longer accepts insurance and is paid an annual fee of about $1,500-$2,000. Some practices charge more, but it is not clear to me what their value could be. Their presence has tarred the term "concierge medicine" with the assumption that it is always expensive. In most cases, the PCP agrees to reduce his or her practice to about 400-500 patients (from the usual 2,500) and give each patient whatever time is necessary. This includes office visits within 24 hours of a call; visiting the patient in the emergency room, hospital or nursing home; and use of email and 24/7 access via the doctor's personal cell phone. An extensive annual evaluation and basic laboratory tests are also included. Of course, if the PCP expects a $1,500-$2,000 annual fee, then the PCP must offer exceptional service. This starts with the receptionist at the front desk, who is now sometimes called a customer service representative, which emphasizes that this first contact person must set the proper tone for the entire experience. Now that the patient pays directly, he or she has every right to expect superior service. Given the emphasis on health and wellness rather than just episodic medical care, this might be termed a "lifestyle" practice model. That said, many of the membership "blue collar" plans described previously offer a large amount of preventive care as well. It only makes economic sense since a healthy patient requires less attention.

The usual justification for the higher retainer fee of $1,500-$2,000 is that the number of patients is lower at 500 than other practices that maintain closer to 800. With fewer patients, the doctor must charge a higher retainer to have the same income as someone who has more patients. One of my PCP interviewees, Dr. Kevin Carlson, is a graduate of a prestigious medical school who completed her residency at an equally well-regarded teaching hospital. She was considered by peers as superb. Dr. Carlson told me that she always wanted to be a high-quality, compassionate physician but found under the old system that she was run ragged, not as thorough as she wanted to be, and had far too little time with her husband and children. She switched to a direct pay approach, accepted no insurance, and reduced her patient number to about 500. After a few months, she told me that she now felt she gave the level of care that her patients deserved. "Before, I thought I was going to die, literally, if I kept this up. I could not give the type of care and attention that I felt was best for my patients. I could not be compassionate. All the things I treasured doing as a doctor had vanished." Talking to one of her patients who had her first annual exam with this PCP under the new system, the patient told me that she "had a new doctor." "Really, did Dr. Carlson bring on a new partner?" "No, it just seemed like a new doctor because she actually listened to me. We had 45 minutes together instead of the former 15 or less. It made a real difference and we actually reviewed all of my issues and questions. I left fully satisfied."

Later Dr. Carlson decided to switch to the retainer approach, charging an annual fee rather than a fee per visit. Setting a limit of 500 patients, she mostly kept the same patients who decided that the level of care improved. After a few years into this new approach, I talked to her again. "The words that I told you on the phone years ago are shocking to me now. I haven't felt that way in so long. I had forgotten how bad I felt before I changed my practice. It has brought tears to my eyes remembering how bitter and resentful I had become. I am embarrassed and humbled by the transformation. I am grateful that I was able fall in love all over again with the practice of medicine. I am doing the job I was born to do, the way I know it should be done. It saddens me that I am in the minority of practicing primary care physicians with high job satisfaction."

Dr. Carlson and others who practice the membership/retainer approach generally give out their personal cell phone numbers and tell their patients to call whenever necessary. Does being essentially "on call" all the time wear the doctor out? Doesn't he or she need time off? My interviews suggest that doctors in these types of practices only receive calls when it is important. Even if they are at a medical meeting out of town, it is often easier to deal with the patient's needs by phone rather than shunting them off to another "covering" physician. As another physician told me, "I have my patients 'trained' to call when they need to but not when it can easily wait until tomorrow morning. If they have an issue, I encourage them to call this evening while we are both still awake rather than wait until 2 a.m. and then realize that the problem has not gone away. That is better for both of us. Very often, I can institute a decision without the need for the patient to come to the office. That saves the patient time and energy and is especially valuable to the person with a chronic illness or two – not only in saving him or her time but in getting care promptly. In the old system, I would have asked him or her to come to the office since I could not get reimbursed by the insurer unless I had a formal face-to-face office visit. "

Switching from a fee-for-service insurance to a direct primary care model (in any of its iterations) can be difficult. One group that attempted the transition a few years ago was pushed back by the state's insurance commissioner. They sent out letters to their patients, set a start date and solicited and collected the annual retainer. There were negative responses from patients, including letters to the editor of the local newspaper saying the doctors were "greedy." A month before the new practice start date, the commissioner informed them that the arrangement essentially offered insurance, which would require an insurance license with regulations and a hefty fee. According to his logic, they offered unlimited primary care services for a single payment, which meant patients would use more or fewer services than others, as with typical insurance. "We were not permitted to 'retain the retainer' and had to refund the checks." During the course of a few years, they were able to reach a compromise with the commissioner, but it was a difficult period for both doctors and patients. Ultimately, they set limits in the new plan on how many visits a person could have per year before requiring an added payment per visit. It was an unfortunate ruling by the commissioner, in my view, but it is a road block that PCPs are encountering in this transformation, which is disruptive to all concerned.[76]

Membership and Hybrid Models that Combine Insurance Reimbursement and Direct Primary Care

Not all physicians are comfortable with completely eliminating insurance. Although the term "direct primary care" implies renunciation of insurance, Concierge Medicine Today reports that perhaps 40 percent of DPC practices actually still take insurance or perhaps some insurance. Under one type of membership model, the practice continues to accept insurance and charges a monthly or annual fee for services not provided by insurance. These might include email, phone consultations, Skype, and additional preventive health time. Although not universal, most physicians in these types of plans reduce their patient panel size to 700-1,000 individuals or fewer. Under this model, you get to know your doctor better, have shorter waits for appointments and have visit times as long as needed.

Some practices are hybrid. They allow patients who wish to join the membership/retainer program to do so, and others remain in the standard model. Those who are members are allowed to use the added benefits, but the remainder, are not. This model is hard to manage. If a non-member patient has a problem, will the PCP say he can only have 10-12 minutes, whereas the other patient gets 25 minutes? It is difficult, at best. The concept of "you get what you pay for" is likely to lead to some hard feelings and loss of patient satisfaction.

Lifestyle and Membership Model Combined Practice

MDVIP Inc. is a form of membership model that puts a heavy emphasis on wellness and lifestyle factors in addition to routine medical care. MDVIP was founded by physicians in 2000, purchased by Procter & Gamble in 2009 and sold to Summit Partners in 2014. As of early 2014, there were more than 700 affiliated PCPs from 42 states and the District of Columbia in the MDVIP network with about 215,000 patients. The PCP is affiliated but not employed by MDVIP. PCPs tend to use this model for the extra security of having an organization behind them to advise on the conversion process, assist in the conversion, address potential legal issues and ensure adequate cash flow, especially in the first year or two. Some feel MDVIP also offers them value by arranging discounted laboratory testing, marketing,

and assistance in finding centers of excellence to refer their patients for complicated issues. The PCP still bills the insurance carrier for routine visits
but also requires a $1,500-$2,200 annual fee, of which one-third goes to
MDVIP for the various services provided to the PCP. He or she limits the
practice to about 600 patients and generally follows the retainer-based practice approach. The PCP includes an extensive preventive medicine annual
exam, including vision, hearing, pulmonary function, an electrocardiogram
if appropriate, a survey of dietary habits, psychosocial issues, and a large battery of blood and urine tests, all as part of the annual fee. The patient meets
with the nurse for about 30 minutes for the testing and blood work about a
week before the annual evaluation. The PCP then spends about 90 minutes
to two hours on the actual exam, review of results and consultation. MDVIP
has a web site with useful information and sends out a newsletter quarterly.
MDVIP doctors also provide access to extensive personalized genetic testing,
cardiovascular assessments and a personalized wellness program.

Does switching to DPC mean a big pay increase for the PCP? Actually,
no. Once office expenses are deducted, along with malpractice and other
costs, the PCP usually ends up with an income akin to what most earned
before, depending on the local demographics.

With about 600 patients (often much less), there is time to actually stop
and think about issues that arise, as in this case of an MDVIP-affiliated doctor who had a relatively new patient with a long history of ITP. Idiopathic
thrombocytopenic purpura is a disease with an unknown cause that diminishes the body's platelets, the particles in the blood stream that prevent
bleeding. Among the accepted treatments are to remove the spleen and to
take corticosteroids. "He was seeing a well-regarded hematologist, had been
treated over the years with splenectomy and now was on steroids. He was
also taking two drugs for high blood pressure. When he came in one day for
a routine visit, his blood pressure was fine but his platelet count was 20,000.
(Normal is about 150,000, and much below 20,000 is the level at which
bleeding is likely to occur.) He had bruises on his legs and told me that he
had to be careful brushing his teeth. If I was still in my old practice, I would
have just told him to see the hematologist, quickly. But now I had some
time. Somewhere in the back of my mind I recalled that a certain thiazide
diuretic could on occasion lower the platelet count. I left the exam room and

looked it up. Sure enough, the drug he was taking had been reported, albeit very uncommonly, to affect platelets. I stopped that medication. Two weeks later his platelet count was 80,000. The hematologist had never considered that possibility. It was only because I had some time to think, to ponder."

How did MDVIP settle on 600 patients? According to an interview with then CEO Dan Hecht, based on data that each patient would get a 1.5 to two-hour annual evaluation, plus an average of three half-hour visits each year (with some needing fewer and some needing more), this leads to a maximum of 600. They have an extensive methodology to transition a physician from the traditional primary care practice to an MDVIP practice. This includes a letter sent to each patient in the PCP's panel and a number of open "town hall" meetings to explain why the change, what it will mean to doctors and patients alike, and what it will cost. An MDVIP staff member essentially "camps" at the PCP's office for about 16 weeks to answer questions and assist with the registration process. To counter the argument that non-registered patients will be left with no physician, or "patient abandonment," MDVIP does not accept a doctor into its program unless analysis shows there are sufficient other PCPs in the area to pick up those not interested in joining the MDVIP model. All of these steps help the PCP work with his or her patients during the transition. Interestingly, although the average PCP has about 2,500 or more patients in the panel, the policy is not "first come, first served" to reach the limit of 600 patients. Instead, usually only about 300 to 350 actually sign up in the first year, with more coming on board via word of mouth over time.

Although there is great variation, most doctors who join with MDVIP are advanced in their careers and find they are getting burned out by "the treadmill" and the lack of enjoyment and satisfaction in their current practice arrangement. It is rare for a doctor just out of training to join because they do not have the large base of patients to draw upon to support the smaller number that will flow to the retainer-based approach.

MDVIP-affiliated doctors, as with most DPC physicians in general, state that they now can delve into the psychosocial issues that underlie many trips to the doctor. For example, one doctor talked about a patient with many difficult-to-control chronic conditions over the years. Nearing the end of the annual evaluation and having developed a closer relationship with his patient, he asked, "Is there anything else we should discuss?" "Well, yes, I was raped in the concentration camp. I never told anyone before just now." With that startling revelation, the doctor was able to finally understand the basis for many of her symptoms and illness problems and was able to rethink the best approaches to her care. He felt that this came about only because he had been able to develop trust as a result of deep nonjudgmental listening rather than rushing the process as he had done in the past.

Reducing Total Costs Through Direct Primary Care

There is limited data about how effective various forms of direct primary care can be in improving quality and reducing costs. Almost all DPC physicians say anecdotally that their new practice approach means the need for fewer specialist referrals, less testing, fewer prescriptions and better overall care quality. But actual studies of DPC efficacy are in short supply. MDVIP is large enough that it can delve into its database for some useful answers. Some argue that MDVIP-affiliated practices are not true DPC since they also accept insurance. True, but the key element is that these PCPs have a reduced patient panel and offer more time with the patient. This makes them useful practices to study. In studies of utilization, patients in MDVIP practices have a rather dramatic drop in hospitalizations, including a 79 percent drop for Medicare enrollees and a 72 percent reduction for those ages 35-64. Elective, non-elective, emergent, urgent, avoidable and unavoidable admissions to the hospital were all lower for the MDVIP members. MDVIP calculates that this saved about $300 million per year in decreased admissions to the hospital, or $2,551 per capita.

Medicare has appropriately put a great emphasis on reducing hospital readmission rates, such as an unplanned readmission to the hospital within 30 days of discharge. Just as admissions of MDVIP patients have fallen, readmissions have declined dramatically. Retrospective review data suggests that the MDVIP patients are more likely to have a variety of preventive measures taken than are those in regular primary care practices. For example, blood pressure control was better, diabetic HbA1c levels (a measure of long term control of blood sugar) were lower, and cholesterol levels were lower. In addition, a higher percentage of patients had mammograms and colonoscopies, as appropriate for sex and age, than the national averages.[77] No data related to perceptions of wellness exists, but the anecdotal information from testimonials have been highly positive.[78]

Qliance is another membership-based practice located in the Northwest with six clinics and roughly 45,000 patients. Their concept was to "stop wasting money" on transaction costs, work for the patient and not the insurer, give providers the time needed to give exemplary care, be open when most convenient for patients (early, late and weekends), and not have incentives to "do stuff." Each doctor has about 800 patients and 10-12 appointments per day. They make extensive use of a team approach and electronic medical records. They also have on-site imaging, basic labs and first-fill drug dispensary, and they obtain pre-negotiated discounted rates for external care when needed by their patients. The monthly fee is a flat $49-$89 based on age. They have found that this model, when combined with a high-deductible insurance plan, saves individuals 20-50 percent per year yet offers comprehensive care while increasing patient (and doctor) satisfaction with better care parameters.

Qliance finds that it spends about two to three times more time per visit, and patients have twice as many visits per year than before. This approach has resulted in a 50 percent decrease in benchmarks for downstream care – 65 percent fewer ER visits, 35 percent fewer hospitalizations, 66 percent fewer specialist visits and 82 percent fewer surgeries. Rather striking results. Qliance estimates that in fee-for-service practices, the average monthly per capita expenditure is $31 for primary care, another $9 for insurer/payer primary care transaction costs, and $290 for all non-primary care, totaling $330 per month. With their comprehensive direct primary care medical home model, the cost for primary care is doubled at $64 per month with no transaction costs and an estimated $194 for all non-primary care, or $254 total. In other words, the Qliance model costs more for primary care but is only about three-quarters of the total cost for the fee-for-service comparative patients.

More recently, Qliance has started to work with large employers, union healthcare trust funds, Medicaid managed care, and a health benefit exchange plan by accepting payment for these groups on the patient's behalf. Even with this arrangement, they have been able to deliver significant savings (10-30 percent lower overall costs net of their charges) with outstanding patient satisfaction scores (>95 percent on almost all of the Agency for Healthcare Research on Quality surveys known as Consumer Assessment of Healthcare Providers and Systems measures or CAHPS).[79]

An analysis done by Qliance management and published in January, 2015[80] found the following among 4,000 Qliance patients covered by employer benefit plans and compared that with non-covered patients who worked for the same employers:

Qliance Savings Data Published January, 2015				
	Incidents Per 1000 Qliance patients	Incidents Per 1000 Non-Qliance patients	Difference (Qliance vs. Other)	Savings Per Patient Per Year
ER Visits	81	94	-14%	($5)
Inpatient Days	100	250	-60%	$417
Specialist Visits	7497	8674	-14%	$436
Advanced Radiology	310	434	-29%	$82
Primary Care Visits	3109	1965	+58%	($251)
Savings per Patient	-	-	-	$679
Total Savings per 1000 patients (after Qliance Fees)				$679,000
Per Cent Saved Per Patient				19.6%

Note that the number of primary care visits are up substantially (58%), but not represented in the chart is the added length of each visit, further adding to the total time spent between patient and doctor.

Iora Health, to be discussed in detail in a later chapter, has found a 13 percent total decline in expenditures, driven primarily by a 37 percent reduction in hospital days, 41 percent decline in hospital admissions, 23 percent decrease in procedures and 48 percent drop in ER visits.

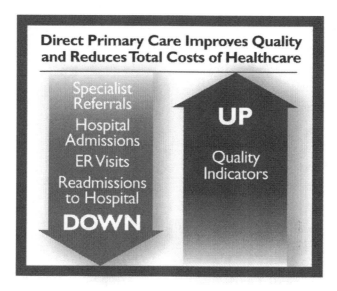

In each of these examples, the key was the PCP-to-patient ratio, more time with the patient, close patient-to-doctor contact by phone and email, and a proactive approach to care, including the use of a team-based approach and health coaches.

Membership and Retainer Practices – For the Elite Only?

A common criticism of membership or retainer-based practices is the added expense. "It is for the elite." Another way to think about the cost is to prioritize expenditures. AtlasMD's annual fee is $600 for a young adult and $1,440 for a family of four. Dr. Neuhofel's fee is $360-$480 annually for an individual and $1,200 for a family. The Izbicki brothers charge $780 per year per individual. As Jon Izbicki puts it, "Our monthly fee is less than what it costs to rent a parking space downtown for the month." Even the more expensive retainer practices are within reason for many. A $1,500 fee is about $4 per day, and $2,000 is about $5.50. How many people spend that much per day at Starbucks – an admittedly pleasant experience but hardly essential? Or consider the monthly/annual cost of a smartphone data contract with AT&T or Verizon Wireless. According to the *Wall Street Journal*[81] and a Department of Labor study, the average American family spends $2,237 per year for the Internet, TV and telephone services. So perhaps $1,500 or $2,000 is not an onerous expense when thinking in terms of prioritizing healthcare expenses relative to other expenses. Of course, it is an *added expense* above and beyond the insurance you already have. But if you have a high-deductible plan with a health savings account (HSA), you can pay for the retainer with tax-advantaged dollars and save considerably compared to a typical insurance policy – plus you will get better care. If you have no insurance, a DPC membership may cost less than using the local urgent care center.

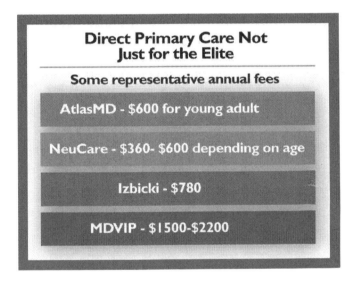

Here is an example of what the tradeoffs in cost might be if you are a 55-year old male or female living in Maryland. The premiums vary by age, but the example here is illustrative for any age group.

The newly-formed insurance exchanges mandated by the Affordable Care Act provide insurers the opportunity to present their policies in a standardized manner so individuals can readily compare plans both within one insurance company and among each of the participating insurance companies. The ACA created four levels, ranging from Bronze with the highest deductible but lowest premium to Platinum with no deductible yet the highest premiums. There are intermediate plans labelled Silver and Gold. Consider a CareFirst (the local Maryland not-for-profit Blue Cross/Blue Shield) policy that provides each of the four levels. In our example, if you choose a Bronze plan for calendar year 2014, the deductible would be $6,000 and the annual premium $3,660 with no copays. If you chose the Platinum plan, there would be no deductible and the premium would be $7,728 per year with maximum hospital copays of $2,000.

Here it is again in a tabular form:

	Bronze	Platinum
Deductible	$6000	$0
Premium (annual)	$3660	$7728
Hospital Co-pay	$0	$2000
Total Maximum Annual Expenses	$9660	$9728

If choosing the high-deductible plan, you could establish a Health Savings Account (HSA) and use those dollars to pay for out-of-pocket expenses, including a DPC membership/retainer. Assuming you were in the 25 percent federal income tax bracket and the 8 percent Maryland bracket for a total of 33 percent, then the after-tax cost to purchase the policy would be just under $2,500 and a $1,500 retainer would be $1,000 for a total of $4,000. (If you were not allowed to pay for the policy with HSA dollars, then you would still save $500 on the retainer.)You could now avail yourself of a direct pay, membership or retainer-based physician who cares for only 500-600 patients and gives unlimited time to each patient, along with cell phone 24/7. Perhaps the comprehensive primary care received would result in better health, fewer illnesses and limited need for added medical services. This is a much better deal than the Platinum plan, which costs more and includes a doctor who gives you 10-12 minutes per visit.

I predict that, absent a significant change in insurer behavior, these retainer-based or direct pay approaches will likely become commonplace in the future of primary care payment. In each of them, it means that you as a patient will obtain real assistance to prevent chronic illnesses from occurring, obtain episodic care for the issues that pop up during the year, receive careful care of your chronic illnesses, and have thorough coordination of the care of chronic illnesses. This will be at a reasonable cost, transparent and with a PCP who has the time to listen – and to listen deeply. I will also predict that the direct primary care retainer-based approaches will blossom into full population health practices over time. Of course, many others disagree with me and believe that DPC will only be a niche practice approach.

In these direct primary care membership/retainer plans with a personal physician-patient contract, market forces will mean that patients will gravitate to the doctor who offers the greatest quality, including time spent with the patient, easy access to office visits and a responsive attitude within a healing environment. The doctor who provides real relationship-based medical care and serves as your "complex care physician" will be successful.

Of course, many of you who already have insurance that covers primary care – commercial or Medicare – might argue that these various direct primary care models represent an added expense, not a savings. You would be correct, but as I have described, the savings can actually be quite substantial. Given the perceived added expense, patients with insurance will only gravitate to these approaches if they find that the quality is substantially greater. Since both physicians and patients are "voting with their feet and checkbooks" and migrating toward these approaches, this suggests that these are becoming considered valid and valuable models for the future.

Those who have no insurance – for whatever reason – will find that they can obtain good quality primary care at a reasonable price from one of the direct pay or membership practices. Perhaps Medicare and Medicaid will decide that it makes sense to pay the retainer and ensure that their enrollees get superior primary care at a reasonable cost while saving Medicare and Medicaid enormous total dollars. We will look at a few plans where this is the case in a later chapter.

This concept applies equally to commercial insurers who, to date, have avoided paying the retainer but should consider it. More often, when asked, they suggest that the employer pay the retainer. At a minimum, the insurer should consider the DPC payment by the patient as counting toward the deductible.

What about employers? Many are converting their health insurance policies to high deductibles, often as high as $10,000 per person or family per year. For a family with members who have chronic illnesses, the costs of healthcare are substantial with these types of deductibles. Employees feel that their employer has walked away from them and saddled them with costs that they simply cannot bear. The company can offset the inherent anger this generates among its employees by paying the retainer for a practice that commits to a low number of total patients, population-style preventive care, and a commitment to developing a close, compassionate relationship with each patient. It is especially valuable for the individual with multiple chronic illnesses since quality primary care can mean much better health and fewer tests, prescriptions, specialist referrals and hospitalizations. I suspect that employers will be the major reason for retainer-based practice growth in the coming years because they will demand that level of service for their staff; more on this in Chapter 17.

I frequently hear the lament that when a PCP converts to direct primary care, many patients get left out, or the "patient abandonment" idea mentioned earlier in the chapter. Some suggest that it may be unethical for the physician to downsize. In describing a hypothetical physician who contemplated converting to DPC, Martinez and Gallagher, writing in the *American Medical Association Journal of Ethics* wrote: "At first blush, this arrangement appears to benefit both doctors and patients. After all, who would object to longer visits, improved access, and enhanced coordination of care? ... Medicine is a profession characterized by fiduciary duties that do not apply to ordinary business practices. A fiduciary relationship acknowledges the imbalance of power between physicians and patients, given the specialized knowledge that physicians possess and the vulnerability associated with being sick. Therefore, unlike commercial interactions in which both parties are expected to act in their own interests, physicians are expected to put patients' interests above their own... Thus, [this physician's] transition practice may result in discontinuity for the majority of her patients, who will have to find new physicians to care for them. The decreased panel size of retainer physicians must be compensated for by other physicians who may already be overburdened, given current shortages in the primary care workforce."[82]

I find this a false argument. To be sure, medicine has a strong ethical background that must be maintained. The physician must always put the patient first. Consider that the 2,500 patients in a typical practice today are not getting superior care. It is the production line approach akin to the *I Love Lucy* segment at the beginning of this chapter. Yes, if many PCPs converted all at once, there could be a serious shortage. But that is not likely to happen. More likely, it is a gradual conversion process by a few PCPs while others seek employment with the hospital, insurer plans, or corporate entities. The affected patients will be cared for by other doctors in the community who still do production medicine. I agree that there will be a short-term market correction, but there does not seem to be another viable model on the horizon that will deliver better care, retain PCPs as practitioners and concurrently attract medical students into primary care. If in a rural area without other physicians the ethical issue does come into play, the physician should still convert but he or she will clearly need to assure that those patients not staying with the practice have a source of care. Perhaps the community will need to rally to recruit another PCP, PA or NP.

PCPs build attachments to their patients over the years. While converting to a practice with fewer patients has all the attractions described, most PCPs are hesitant to do so. They simply do not want to have to face their patients and say, "You cannot all come with me to my new practice." Some patients will say "no." As one patient wrote in response to one of my blog posts, "DPC will actually be an abbreviation for 'Dumped by Primary Care.'" It is a conundrum for many and will remain so until patients begin to appreciate the value of comprehensive care and demand it.

Once it becomes clear that people like you can receive better care at a reasonable cost, you and your neighbors will be the ones who will pressure PCPs to make the conversion. It is supply and demand. If the demand is there, the supply will increase. Direct primary care is one way to fix the system.

The alternative is to wait and let the doctor burn out and close his or her practice, in which case no one receives the benefit of that doctor. The current high visit number is a direct consequence of a reimbursement system that has paid too little for too long. If that had never happened, there would never have been the pressure to see too many patients or have too large a panel size. The need today is to return to a reasonable number of visits per day. Using better technology and team functions, that number can be somewhat greater today than it was years ago, but it still needs to be a reasonable number that the PCP can interact with appropriately. Plus, doctors today spend an inordinate time on nonclinical (and probably mostly non useful) paperwork. Direct primary care gives at least 20 percent of that time back.

As medical students begin to observe that it is possible to be a high quality PCP who gives superior care in a satisfying setting, more will once again choose to become PCPs.

Consider this comment by Dr. Joel Bessemer, a DPC internist in Omaha, Nebraska: "To those who say concierge doctors are hurting the system by diminishing the number of patients we can care for, my reply is: If you keep doing the same thing year after year, you are going to get the same results. If we don't focus on salvaging the doctor-patient relationship and allowing the appropriate time for each patient's care and follow-up, patients will begin to feel their primary care is a waste of time."[83]

That is the same idea a neighbor of mine said when his doctor decided to transition to DPC. This patient felt that his PCP was of little importance. He received most of his care from his cardiologist and his urologist, so why did he even need the PCP? Frankly, he did not, given the former practice model. But he would benefit from a PCP who could offer him the time he really needed – time that would mean better care and fewer visits to the specialists. He remained unconvinced and went without a PCP for the next few years. His wife, however, did make the switch and, being pleased with the new arrangement, prodded her husband to join a few years later. He still grouses about the retainer but is pleased with the care he now receives.

Consider this analogy, as told to me by Dr. Josh Umbehr of AtlasMD. Think of PCPs as light bulbs. If you overload them, they burn out. Right now the bulbs (PCPs) are burning out from overload. Direct primary care is like setting the bulb to 60 watts and keeping it there. It can function well for a long time. A longer burn with more net light is equivalent to a long productive career with patients receiving expanded primary care. Since it is comfortable to burn at 60 watts, we are likely to see more light bulbs produced – or more medical students choosing primary care again.

Dr. Izbicki told me, "DPC is a business model ....that holds both the doctor and patient accountable within a transparent system." I call this balancing rights with responsibilities by both doctor and patient.

Dr. Horvitz suggested, "Hopefully as DPC becomes more mainstream and accepted, it can become the norm for primary care and patients will realize that this is the [best] model. When that occurs the shortage of primary care physicians will end as primary care will once again become more popular among medical students and residents.... It is a rare patient in my practice who over utilizes my time or the system. They just want time and access."

Primary care does not need to be expensive. Paradoxically, the insurance methodology has made it so. In the direct pay and retainer/membership models, the physician and the patient generally break the bonds with the insurer and replace it with a direct contractual relationship with each other. The upfront cost per capita of primary care is more, but the result is more time for each patient, which results in much better care, greater satisfaction for the patient and doctor and reduced overall healthcare costs. Frustrations go way down. We need to appreciate that the PCP's life will be better, and health and wellness will be more accessible, improving medical care. With more time for each patient, there will be fewer stories of rushed and inadequate care, like the one of Susan that began this book.

CHAPTER FIFTEEN

INNOVATORS: INURANCE PROVIDERS WHO GOT IT RIGHT

Insurance payments to primary care physicians have been so low for such a long time that there is now a shortage of PCPs. But a number of insurers have "seen the light" and are developing new approaches to primary care that improve quality and reduce overall costs.

Fee-for-Service with an Increased Insurance Reimbursement – Incenting the PCP

CareFirst Blue Cross Blue Shield believed that good care coordination would improve the quality of care for the individual patient with a chronic illness and reduce costs by eliminating excess visits, tests, and procedures. With that the assumption, CareFirst instituted a new program that incents PCPs with opportunities for increased income in return for providing effective chronic illness care coordination and enhanced preventive care. This is another example of balancing rights with responsibilities on the part of both parties. More than three years into the program, the results are clear: care is improved, patient and PCP satisfaction has improved, and the savings in total costs of care have been reduced – all with fewer referrals to specialists and reduced hospitalizations.

CareFirst has the largest market share for commercial (for example, under age 65) health insurance in its region at 40 percent. CareFirst calculates that about 65 percent of their medical expenditures go toward the care of just 5 percent of patients, and 80 percent of expenditures cover about 15 percent. These are patients with complex chronic illnesses. CareFirst also knows that primary care physicians receive about 5 percent of total healthcare expenditures, yet they are in a position to strongly impact much of the other 95 percent. CareFirst also wants to raise awareness of healthy lifestyles to assist their enrollees to remain healthy. The CareFirst agenda was to create incentives for PCPs to reduce the total cost for those with chronic conditions and maintain the health of the remaining enrollees. This latter approach effectively makes the plan a population health approach, in addition to the care of those with chronic illnesses.

This is how the plan works: PCPs form into actual or virtual groups of 5 to 10 and enter into an agreement with CareFirst. CareFirst increases their reimbursement by 12 percent for each visit. CareFirst agrees to pay the physician within one business day, dramatically reducing the doctor's need for working capital.

CareFirst does an actuarial analysis of the PCP group's patients by using claims data from the prior year to create an anticipated "global budget" for the coming year. CareFirst is able to "flag" the 15 percent of patients who need care coordination. The PCP's obligation in this new system is to give the patient whatever added time is needed per visit, create a good care plan and post it in an electronic medical record, for which the PCP receives an additional $200. This serves as automatic preauthorization, and no further calls to CareFirst are needed for tests, procedures, or imaging. This is another major time saver for the PCP and office staff. The concept also anticipates that with extra time per patient, the PCP can handle most issues, even patients with complex chronic illnesses. When the patient needs to see a specialist, the PCP refers the patient but also calls the specialist to clarify expectations and review the results of the referral when done. Finally, CareFirst makes available a nurse "care coordinator" at CareFirst's expense to call the patient as often as necessary to check on medication use, medication side effects, blood pressure, blood glucose levels, weight gain or other aspects of the patient's care plan. If the care coordinator cannot resolve an issue or sees a developing problem, she reports it to the PCP. The expectation starting out was that this incentive approach would enhance quality yet reduce the overall expenditures for patients with chronic illnesses.

If the PCP group's total claims come in under the projected global budget at the end of the year, CareFirst gives back a portion of the savings through even higher reimbursements. With these incentives, they anticipate that the PCP would carefully coordinate care so there are no excess specialist visits, no unneeded tests or procedures and fewer hospitalizations. The end result would be higher quality care, lower total expenditures, higher income for the PCPs and a more satisfying practice. It could be a win for everyone. Now a few years in, the plan seems to be working. The physicians are pleased with the added income, CareFirst is pleased that total costs have dropped, and presumably, the patients are pleased that they are getting better care.

The care coordination described above is a major part of the new CareFirst plan. But there are other important components of the plan. The PCP receives increased compensation for all of his or her CareFirst patients, not just those with complex chronic illness. This might ensure that every patient receives the time and attention needed for the best possible care. It also means that the PCP is less inclined to quickly refer a patient to a specialist rather than take the time needed. It also encourages the physician to do a more complete history and physical exam, negating the need for more tests and procedures. The result is better care for the patient, a more satisfied patient who does not feel "rushed" and a more satisfied physician. Once again, the goal is better care at lower total cost.

CareFirst recognizes that more than 90 percent of their clients remain with them year after year, so it is financially logical to ensure good preventive care. This costs more today but should pay off in the years to come with lower costs as the patient remains healthy. In this new practice arrangement, CareFirst pays for any preventive program or screening test that is well defined by evidence. This might include cholesterol measurements, mammography and colonoscopy, dietary consultation, or a smoking cessation program. As an added incentive to seek this type of preventive care, CareFirst waives any co-pays or deductibles that the patient might have to otherwise pay. The Affordable Care Act has done the same for policies purchased within the exchanges and now requires all insurers to waive deductibles and co-pays for preventive care.

Finally, CareFirst recognizes that a small percentage of patients will develop a catastrophic condition that the PCP can no longer easily coordinate. These are the 5 percent of patients who consume a large portion of healthcare dollars. This is the patient who must be referred to a specialty center or an academic medical center, have major surgery or receive an organ transplant. Based on my observations over the years, these are the patients who receive less than the best care because the referrals among providers – even within the same hospital – are less than satisfactory. This is where quality breaks down, safety issues arise, and excess tests and procedures happen. Since no one orchestrates the entire care program, the patient is left with well-intentioned caregivers but less than the best care. [The nearby graphic is adapted from an article in *Health Affairs* by Susan Dentzer interviewing CareFirst CEO Chet Burrell, see reference 82]

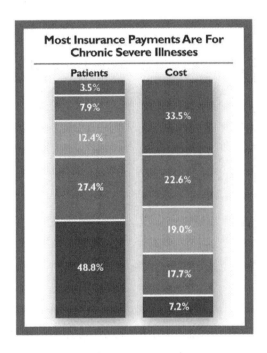

In this situation, CareFirst develops an incentive-based relationship with the specialty provider – probably a hospital system – to ensure care coordination. The hospital system assigns a "navigator" to each patient. The navigator makes sure the care of the patient within the system is well coordinated, just as the PCP does in the community setting. This navigator works the interface among the myriad specialists, departments, hospitals and centers that the patient must utilize for his or her care. CareFirst postulates that there could be better quality yet at a substantially reduced total cost.[84]

The overall concept is to coordinate patient care with the expectation that the patient will be better served, the providers will be more satisfied and the total costs will be reduced.[85] It means a transformation in how the PCP functions – a change from being an intervener to also being an orchestrator. It is a significant change for the hospital as well, which, in an era of fee-for-service, means less revenue. It is also a huge transformation for the insurer – a change that was initially resisted within CareFirst. It is a change that accepts that extensive primary care with care coordination costs money but recognizes that the end result is better quality at a lower cost.

After two years, CareFirst reported that it saved $136 million with 297 panels of 3,600 PCPs who joined the program and cared for about one million individuals. All of the PCPs enjoyed the added income to their reimbursements, and two-thirds received end-of-year incentive payments sufficient to represent a total increase of about 29 percent over CareFirst's then existing fee schedule.[86]

At the end of three years and with enough data to be actuarially credible, there have been definite improvements in 10 measures, such as costs per-member per-month, cost of emergency visits, admissions per 1,000 members, length of stay, cost per admission, and readmissions after discharge within 30 days. Specifically, there have been 6 percent fewer hospital admissions, 11 percent fewer days in the hospital and 11 percent fewer outpatient visits. The PCPs who were most successful were those who spent more time with their patients, referred to specialists less, and when they did, chose specialists who were less inclined to over utilize expensive yet unnecessary testing like CT or MRI scans. Program savings show that the total patient expense growth last year was 3.5 percent, which is the lowest rate in years and means lower premium increases next fall. For those who purchase insurance directly, the savings will be all theirs. For those with insurance via an employer, the savings will be shared by both employer and employee in the form of lower premiums and out-of-pocket costs.

Not all panels of PCPs were as successful as others, and those who were successful tended to be so in each of the three years in the program. At the end of the third year, about 60 percent of the panels were granted an incentive award for beating their projected global budget level by an average of

6.3 percent. The 40 percent that were unsuccessful were above target by an average of 3.9 percent, a spread of almost 10 points. The successful panels tended to be those in small private practices and, interestingly, had sicker patients under care, yet they maintained higher quality scores. The panels composed of PCPs employed by large health systems tended to be among the bottom performers. Those in small private practices were more likely to refer to lower-cost specialists than those who were employed by larger health systems. As I have noted elsewhere, hospital-based PCPs are encouraged to refer internally. It also may be pertinent that the hospital-based PCP often does not personally share in any incentive payment from CareFirst – his or her employer keeps the incentives and pays the PCP based on its own internal contractual relationship.[87]

An additional outcome of this "experiment" was the finding that specialists could be stratified as low, moderate or high-cost relative to similar medical conditions. CareFirst has found there is often a 100 percent variation in the cost of an "episode" of care depending on which specialist was selected. It will be interesting to learn if referral patterns change once this information is disseminated to the PCPs, as is being done this year.

Perhaps the most important outcome is the recognition by a major insurer that it is possible to create a new incentive-based approach to reimbursement – in this case, within the old fee-for-service model – that actually costs more for primary care (up from about 5 percent of total costs to about 7 percent of total costs) yet significantly reduces those total costs of care while improving quality.

A reasonable question is whether these savings benefit the entity paying the premiums (person, employer, union) or just CareFirst. The answer is that if the total costs of care go down or at least do not rise, then the premiums increase little or not at all in the following year. Of course, this becomes a marketing advantage for CareFirst.

After this program was underway, CareFirst obtained an innovation grant to pilot Medicare in their model. Approximately 35,000 enrollees in Traditional Medicare in Maryland participate in this plan, which began January 1, 2014. It follows the same precepts as mentioned above. CareFirst offered this opportunity to a select number of the virtual PCP panels, chosen based on success with the younger patients discussed above. On average, the 14 PCP panels participating in this pilot have about 2,500 CareFirst members under age 65 and now about 2,000 Medicare beneficiaries, for a total annual target budget of about $50 million. The opportunity for shared savings between PCP and CareFirst at this level becomes a powerful motivator for quality care.

Next Step – Incenting the Patient

Having determined which primary care physicians were effective in improving quality, coordinating care and holding down costs, CareFirst will embark on an added program that will encourage its policy holders to utilize one of the highest-ranking PCPs in their network. In return, CareFirst will eliminate co-pays and deductibles for the sickest patients who agree to cooperate with their PCP and comply with the developed care plans.

Using Medicare Advantage to Improve Primary Care for the Elderly

Older individuals have more health concerns and more complex chronic illnesses, along with impaired vision, hearing, mobility and cognition. Older individuals consume far more medical resources and dollars than the remainder of the population. These individuals are benefitted with more intense primary care, attendant preventive care, close disease monitoring and attention to chronic illness.

A Medicare Advantage Plan called Erickson Advantage through United Healthcare includes only residents of Erickson Living continuing care retirement communities and sets the patient number per doctor at a remarkably low 400 for their in-house PCPs. They found that 400 is the ideal number of elderly geriatric residents per doctor in order to ensure a quality, humanistic, integrative approach to care. The PCPs do not act alone but rather lead a team based medical home that includes NPs, RNs, social workers and others. Residents enjoy rapid access to the PCP, resident-centered care, engagement of the residents, an approach that plans and manages care in an integrated fashion and utilizes an electronic medical record. Erickson Living wants their residents to be independent and be well to the degree possible and to that aim they try to deliver expert comprehensive and personalized health and wellness services, not just "medical care." They have clearly demonstrated that this approach to primary care with a low number of patients per doctor and a team effort not only gives superior care but also results in reduced total costs of health care. In the Erickson plans (there are five to choose from based on personal situations and circumstances), a patient can continue to use a community PCP or choose the on-site PCPs, access a wide range of specialists when necessary (many conduct office hours on site), use almost any hospital, and receive a ride to most off-site doctors' offices at no cost. Under Traditional Medicare, a patient must spend three days in the hospital (admitted, not under observation – a critical difference) in order to be eligible for Medicare to pay for the first 100 days of residential skilled nursing care. But this Advantage plan waives the required three-day stay. The doctor can make the decision and arrange immediate referral to their on-campus site. This eliminates a costly hospitalization. The plan has an on-site nurse to coordinate special needs, such as preparing for surgery, returning to the community from the hospital, transferring to assisted living, and arranging in-home special needs care. There is also an on-site benefits specialist to assist residents with their questions. In 2014, the most common plan cost $189 per month or $2,268 per year. This is substantially less than one might pay for both Medigap and Part D policies, yet it includes greater benefits (such as basic dental) with few co-pays and no deductibles.

According to medical director Mathew Narrett, MD, residents can have same or next-day appointments for a long as needed, and they are offered extensive preventive care. In addition, the PCPs are well-versed in gerontology issues and have a strong commitment to listening. As part of the resident-centered approach, the resident receives a printed copy of their medical record at the conclusion of each visit. Some of the results of this approach: Chronic illnesses can be managed successfully without the need for referral to specialists, but when needed, specialists are readily available. Hospital admissions are down in comparison to equivalent groups of elderly individuals. The length of stay in the hospital for those who must be admitted is much lower. As noted previously, the 30-day unanticipated readmission rate has consistently been below 11 percent (the national rate is about 20 percent) despite the average age of their residents being about 82.

When referral to a specialist is needed, the PCP will suggest a physician that is fully cognizant of the varying needs of a geriatric population. The PCP's team arranges for the appointment, sends a note to the specialist including the reason for the referral, a problem list and a medication list so that the specialist will be fully informed in advance of the visit. Dr. Narrett explained that one of their guiding principles is to arrange for as much care as possible on site. To this regard, Erickson Living provides space for specialists such as cardiology, orthopedics and dermatology to see patients on campus. Since vision, hearing, foot care and oral care is critical to seniors, they rent space for optometrists, audiologists and dentists and employ a podiatrist.

I have had the opportunity to talk to a resident of one community that had recently fallen and broken his pelvis during the middle of the night. He called the security desk, they responded immediately and determined that he should go to the hospital for X-rays. His physician from the community visited early in the morning already knowing the resident's medical history, medications, etc. from assessing his electronic medical record. After determining that it was a fractured pelvis and not femur, he was discharged to the community's rehabilitation center and upon arriving they knew his issues, what to expect, had his medical record and had his medications laid out (including his over the counter meds such as calcium tablets.) There was no need for someone to go to his apartment, look in his medicine closet and fetch whatever he might need. He told me that he was very satisfied with the care and the care process. Separately, I talked to a large group of residents in another Erickson Living community when I was invited to lecture about advances in medical science. During the Q&A period, and with no Erickson staff present, I asked if there was general satisfaction with the care offered, with the doctors and the staff and with the insurance option. Just about every hand went up in affirmation to each.

My takeaway is that when the PCPs are experts in caring for the elderly and when given the needed time, the care is excellent, satisfaction is strong, and the total costs come down substantially.

Here are some other examples related to older individuals. Humana and Iora Health have recently announced a partnership to provide Medicare Advantage patients in Arizona and Washington with comprehensive primary care using the Iora Health approach. They will begin with two practices in each state exclusively for Humana's Medicare Advantage members and will include not only PCPs but also nurses, health coaches (an integral aspect of all Iora Health endeavors), social workers, mental health experts and others. Since the patients will all be over 65, they will receive care designed for their age group with limited numbers of patients per doctor and team. As with the Erickson retirement communities, this resource-intense approach will cost more for primary care, but the expectation is an accentuation of wellness, improved care coordination, improved patient satisfaction, high quality and reduced costs.

These are just a few examples of how some insurers are changing the paradigm so patients, especially those with complex chronic illnesses, can get better care, including good preventive care and care coordination. Hopefully more insurers will follow suit with multiple innovative approaches so the best can be sorted out in the marketplace.

CHAPTER SIXTEEN

INNOVATORS: PRIMARY CARE-BASED ORGANIZATIONS THAT ARE IMPROVING CARE

Change is mandatory in order to salvage and improve primary care for America. Change needs to be dramatic, not just tinkering around the edges. Where will change come from? One clear answer is from innovative, enthusiastic groups that are committed to reinvigorating primary care. Some are developing grassroots interest and advocacy. Others are establishing new models of care. Here is a selection.

Loss of Clout - From Frustration to Action

Most PCPs – and most other physicians – believe that legislators and other policymakers do not listen to doctors' viewpoints. They feel they are often the only ones who are not consulted. They have strong feelings about the development of the Affordable Care Act and believe that the American Medical Association (AMA) was not sufficiently cognizant or supportive of the PCP's needs. The result, they believe, is that the ACA does not address the payments to PCPs, other than the 10 percent Medicare increase and the temporary Medicaid equivalency directive. It also did not address the issue of malpractice reform. The AMA did work vigorously to have the Medicare Sustainable Growth Rate (SGR) system replaced, but despite the AMA's support of the ACA, the SGR still exists. Additionally, the ACA did little to address either costs or quality – only access. In general, PCPs do not believe a large powerful organization is on their side or advocating for them.

Most physicians avoid the political process but have done so to their ultimate detriment. Plus, the needs of the primary care physician often differ from those of specialists. The American Medical Association was traditionally the political action entity that physicians relied upon to voice their concerns to government, including Congress. About 75 percent of all physicians were members 50 years ago, but today only about 15 percent are members. Primary care physicians see the AMA as not representing them because the organization is largely composed of specialists. Likewise, the American College of Physicians (internists) is largely comprised of specialists. Nevertheless, some PCPs are members of one or both organizations and are attempting to have their voices heard. In addition, the Academy of Family Physicians, which only has PCPs as members, represents a unified voice for primary care.

Primary Care Progress

Now a new crop of young primary care physicians, nurse practitioners, physician assistants and students interested in a primary care career have begun to band together and create new grassroots organizations. One called Primary Care Progress was founded by primary care providers "united by a new vision for revitalizing the primary care workforce pipeline through interprofessional collaboration and strategic local advocacy that promotes primary care and transforms care delivery and training in academic settings." Within a few years of its formation, PCP has accrued more than 3,000 members in 40 chapters, mostly aligned with medical schools. Primary Care Progress attempts transformation with grassroots organizing to empower primary care providers and aspiring students. The national organization supports chapters and individuals with training in advocacy, developing leadership skills and working with the media.

"One of the biggest problems in healthcare is that we've all been operating as lone rangers, trying to fix the variety of problems we face by relying upon ourselves," Andrew Morris-Singer, MD, a founder and president, told me in an interview. "This has been our approach in the clinic as well as in the classroom and in the halls of government. But the problems we face are massive – so big that the only way we'll fix them is if we band together and consolidate our power. Simply put, we've got to team in all domains."

However, adds Morris-Singer, teaming does not come naturally in healthcare. "We need to be incredibly intentional about it. And we need to

ensure that it's an inclusive team, engaging the non-MDs, as well as trainees and patients. That's the only way we'll have the power and influence to
protect our new approach to primary care delivery from being derailed and
destroyed by those who oppose it."

Morris-Singer believes the key to getting patients on board is to improve
the quality of care they receive. "And that's an inherently local process – not
dictated by a policy or cookie-cutter template. But we also need to engage
the patients in the improvement and transformation process. Not just so we
incorporate their needs and preferences. But also so we get them emotionally
invested in us, and our clinics."

For Morris-Singer, all of this comes down to relationships, or politics.
"At PCP, we're teaching the next generation how to start working in a much
more strategic and tactical way. We're building a new generation of primary
care leaders and activists."[88]

Primary Care Action Coalition

This group was initiated by Andy Lazris, MD, a geriatrician who, like so
many full time practicing primary care physicians, is deeply frustrated. Not
by actually caring for patients but at the impediments placed in the path
of good care by the arcane rules and regulations of insurers, notably in his
case by Medicare. He notes that he was a supporter of the ACA but that
with its passage his work and frustration level have only increased. Why?
The EMR adds about an hour or more per day to document so that he is
compliant with "meaningful use" and is not dinged with a reduced Medicare
payment structure. Arranging for home health, a wheelchair or other means
that would allow a patient to be cared for a home rather than in the hospital
is complex and difficult, at best. "Reformers require us adhere to a huge
array of quality indicators, none of which has been demonstrated to reflect
true quality, and all of which leads to unnecessary busy work that detracts
from the care of our patients. Meanwhile, reformers have not tackled the real
drivers of high cost, low quality health care in our system--*an excessive reliance
on hospitalization, specialization, testing, invasive procedures, and medication use.*
[italics mine] Especially for the elderly, home-based palliative care has been
demonstrated to be the most beneficial, cost-effective, and patient endorsed

means of providing medical services, and yet insurances such as Medicare will not pay for such true quality, a reality that has not been addressed in current reform efforts." He also notes that physicians and especially primary care physicians are never consulted when Medicare (or insurers in general) develop their guidelines.

The mission: "PCAC is a consortium of practicing primary care doctors who are advocating for a larger role in health care reform to promote sensible medical care."[89]

It is likely that more groups like Primary Care Progress and Primary Care Action Coalition will develop in the coming years to offer a unified, local and national voice to represent the needs of the PCP – and in the process improve the care of their patients.

Developing an Integrated Approach to Primary Care - Casey Health Institute

Casey Health Institute was founded in Gaithersburg, Maryland, with the philanthropic assistance of Mrs. Betty Casey and the Eugene Casey Foundation. Mrs. Casey engaged husband-and-wife physicians David Fogel and Ilana Bar-Levav to do a six-month look at various models of integrative healthcare across the United States. From this, they developed a plan and received a $30 million grant from the Casey Foundation, along with a fully-renovated 72,000 square foot office building. According to Dr. Fogel, "Our vision is to build a team-based collaborative culture in which people will value and actively engage in their own health and well-being. Our mission is to create a new model of integrative health care, a model that transforms the patient/provider relationship in the context of a non-profit, community-based health center." Although a not-for-profit entity with all staff employed, once the seed money is exhausted, it must still pay its staff through dollars earned from patient care. The Institute is working to advance innovative economic models with the medical models of care.

Up and running since early 2013, the Casey Health Institute has both a primary care practice and a wellness center. The Wellness Center includes preventive medicine and health maintenance as integral aspects of the Institute, with the wellness center available for improving health in body, mind and spirit with exercise, relaxation, meditation, stress control and other modalities. The primary care program incorporates primary care physicians, nurse practitioners, naturopaths, psychologists, chiropractic care, acupuncture, and massage therapy in an integrative manner. Rather than deal principally with episodic care, the Institute practitioners aim to affect health maintenance as a primary objective, not secondary. Each patient has a personal physician or nurse practitioner but is also directly connected to a team of providers based on individual need. According to Dr. Fogel, "By combining integrative medicine with conventional medical primary care, our practice reframes not only how we encourage patients to think about their own health, but also how we, as practitioners, think about how we provide the best care and wellness services to our patients."

A Focus on the Most Medically Needy - AbsoluteCARE

AbsoluteCARE

AbsoluteCARE was established as a an infectious disease practice in Atlanta, initially dedicated to HIV patients but soon expanded to a broad primary care program for those with multiple serious chronic illnesses. It includes the 5 percent of individuals who consume 40-50 percent of all medical dollars. It is a subsidiary of Avesis, a dental, hearing and vision benefits plan operator, and is expanding to other markets. The newest site is in Baltimore, where it recently opened a 17,000 square foot primary care clinic to manage the care of those with chronic illnesses. These include "the sickest of the sick" whose prior year average annual claims approach $80,000 per year or more. Initial health plans that use AbsoluteCARE are a Medicaid managed care plan and a Medicare Advantage plan sponsored by Amerigroup. The model employs one PCP or NP per 300 patients (compared to the usual 2,500+ in most primary care practices) working with a team that includes a case manager, medical assistant and nurse. Other professionals include a therapist, psychiatrist, social worker, and nutritionist. In addition to medical care, they address social issues that impact health status, such as food, clothing, housing and transportation. For example, they transport the patient to and from the clinic, and the nutritionist shops with the patient to address food choices. In short, AbsoluteCARE puts enormous primary care resources at the care disposal of each patient.

The Baltimore clinic is notable for its ambience, cleanliness, courteous staff, and a sense of fun amid the seriousness. The clinic gives off the clear message that everyone cares about the patients and is determined to develop a trusting, healing relationship with each. It is not exactly what one might expect in an inner city medical office that caters to the socioeconomically disadvantaged.

The facility has four "pods," each with sufficient exam rooms for the eight provider teams. The initial visit is no less than an hour, and subsequent visits are no less than 40 minutes – no 10-15 minute appointments. The provider-patient ratio ensures that each patient receives thorough attention, which is warranted given their precarious medical circumstances. A major focus is on the family and social situations: Do they live alone? Do they have transportation? Do they have difficulties paying for rent, phone or heating bills? During each visit, the patient is seen by the case manager, the medical assistant and the doctor/nurse practitioner, and they then hold a team conference after each patient. The case manager then discusses next steps with the patient and establishes an action plan for the patient and the members of the team to accomplish, complete with dates and expected results. The plan may also involve the social worker to help the patient access community social service organizations and address the patient's direct medical needs.

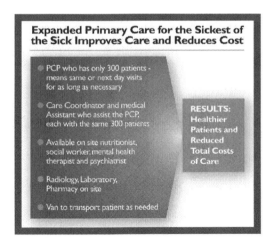

Patients receive appointments immediately upon calling but can also drop in anytime or call their provider. In addition, patients can receive acute treatment such as IV fluids, IV antibiotics, and IV diuresis in the center. There is an in-house lab; special tests can be sent out. Once at full capacity, there will be an in-house pharmacy as well, which will create a higher level of convenience, control and oversight of medications. General radiology is transmitted via the Internet to a nearby tele-radiologist.

AbsoluteCARE has a cadre of specialists who they tend to call on for referrals – chosen not only for their expertise but also for their willingness to work in close coordination with the care team. Should a patient need hospitalization, the social worker interacts with the nearby hospital's social worker and the doctor interacts with the hospitalist. Patients can be admitted directly, bypassing the ER and its attendant costs. At the time of discharge, AbsoluteCARE picks up the patient, brings him or her to the clinic to review discharge instructions, and then takes the patient home. Should a patient be admitted to another hospital, AbsoluteCARE makes every effort to see the patient within 48 hours after discharge, recognizing that to wait any longer will often mean a readmission for these fragile patients.

As the medical director Greg Foti, MD told me, "It is all about vigilance and caring. Our aim is to put the caring back into healthcare, and we are serious about that. Our standards are not how many patients did you see today but how much quality did you dispense today. We must call the hospitalist if the patient is admitted. We must follow-up with skilled nursing if needed. We must transport them here to be sure they actually get the care they need. We want to fully wrap our arms around all the factors that affect their health. We don't have any magic bullets, but we can give true love and care to our 'members.' That will make the difference in both quality and costs."[90]

The fundamental concept is that if the patient receives good primary care in a patient-centered medical home with team-based functions, including attention to social, medical and mental requirements, then they will be much healthier and use fewer medical system resources, especially expensive ER visits, procedures, imaging, specialist visits and hospitalizations. The focus is on complex care and care coordination with a good dose of preventive medicine.

The business model is to receive per-member per-month (PMPM) payments from the insurer (in this case, mostly Medicaid via Amerigroup) for each high-risk patient at a level that supports this resource-intense program. Given that these individuals have multiple extensive chronic illnesses that cannot be cured, it is impossible to drive the costs down toward a typical healthy population, but AbsoluteCARE has demonstrated that costs can been substantially reduced, even with these difficult-to-treat patients. The Atlanta clinic has been effective with a one-third reduction in total healthcare expenses. The Baltimore clinic opened in February 2014, so results are a few years away. With this model, primary care is expensive because extensive resources are placed for the patients' care, but total costs come way down. The beneficiaries are not only the patients but also the taxpayers who support Medicaid. It is another example in which allowing adequate time with the PCP and his or her team can be highly beneficial.

AbsoluteCARE and other organizations that follow this model of placing extensive primary care resources at the benefit of the most expensive patients are doing something similar to that of Dr. Jeffery Brenner in Camden, New Jersey and described by Dr. Atule Gawande.[91] In brief, Brenner, a family physician, studied "hot spots" in the city and soon learned that those for whom the most expenditures were consumed were those that cycled in and out of the hospital and were those who by many standards were receiving the least beneficial care. He then established a clinic that included not only doctors but social workers, nutritionists, behavioral health coaches, etc. and the clinic did its part to assure that patients got to appointments and took their medications. As one measure of success, there was a 40% reduction in hospital and ER visits and a 56% reduction in hospitalization expenses. The moral of the story is that extensive primary care, although more expensive that routine primary care, will markedly improve health while likewise cutting the total costs of care. This is the message that employers, insurers and government officials need to appreciate.

AbsoluteCARE providers and others following a similar model are effectively practicing population health concepts as described in Chapter 8 with their panel of patients. Rather than wait for the patient to call with a problem, the team at AbsoluteCARE is proactively addressing primary (health and wellness promotion), secondary (screening) and tertiary prevention.

For these high risk, high utilizer individuals, most of the effort is directed toward tertiary prevention – working to minimize disease complications and comorbidities.

Other Corporate Approaches to Direct Primary Care

Iora Health

Another company that focuses on the most medically needy is Iora Health. A Boston physician, Rushika Fernandopulle, MD, and a serial entrepreneur, Christopher McKown, established it as a new approach to the concept of relationship-based primary care. As of early 2014, they obtained $20 million in venture seed capital. They sought to redesign primary care from the bottom up rather than "tweaking the existing model. Maybe what we need to do is start from the beginning, from scratch," said Fernandopulle.[92] Each patient has a PCP, a health coach and, via a sponsor, pays a flat, all-inclusive monthly membership fee of about $80 for comprehensive primary care, including educational programs, email, texting, video and a population health approach to follow-ups.

"What we have been doing in this health care system is illogical," says Andrew Schutzbank, MD, M.P.H., assistant medical director of Iora Health and a founding member of Primary Care Progress. "The system is upside down. The key is relationship building, but today primary care can't work because we got rid of the relationship between the PCP and patient. The fee-for-service system reinforces the problem. It pushes the doctor to spend a lot of time doing things that can be documented instead of spending real time in building a relationship with the patient. So we needed to just dispose of the old model and start anew. The old system emphasizes the visit with the doctor, but we know that it is not only possible but often preferable to interact in other ways - ways not covered by current insurance – like email, telephone, Skype or text. We can save the patient time, money and give better care. Often the patient does not need much of our time, but 'they need it when they need it,' and we can respond to that."[93]

One of their key tenets is to help patients better manage their own health and navigate the health care system. Since so much of health depends on behavior, they help with behavioral change as needed through the development of a close relationship between patient and doctor and especially between patient and health coach. The PCPs and health coaches work together, caring for a more manageable panel size. The coach's role is to become close with the patient as a mentor, friend and trusted confidant. As Schutzbank told me "Trust builds from actively accomplishing what the patient needs." Coaches help the patient follow through with the plan set out jointly by the physician and the patient. Coaches also help patients advocate for themselves. The team huddles each morning to discuss the patients scheduled for the day and actions needed as follow-up for patients seen in the past. For example: Did the colonoscopy get scheduled? Was it completed? Are the new blood pressure medications being taken? Are they working? Is the patient having difficulty accessing needed services?

The business model has been to seek insurer, employer or union sponsorship, which in turn pays the PMPM fee. There are no other transactional charges – no co-pays, no deductibles. If the patient needs laboratory work, imaging or medications, IoraHealth finds low-cost providers who accept the patient's underlying insurance.

Iora Health tries to keep a close working relationship with the sponsor or payer. Often, "we are able to convince the sponsor to see the value in paying for things generally not considered part of medical care. That might be cab fare to assure that a patient can get to appointments, an air conditioner to help a patient with asthma, or purchase needed medications that the patient simply cannot afford. All of these help to keep the patient as healthy as possible and, importantly, out of the emergency room or the hospital with its attendant high costs and risks of complications." Schutzbank described a patient that was frequently in the ER and admitted to the hospital, costing tens of thousands of dollars. The sponsor agreed to pay cab fare to get the patient to his Iora Health appointments, and now he is seen regularly and has had a significant decrease in his trips to the ER.

Iora Health began by focusing on the most sick – those with multiple complex, chronic illnesses akin to AbsoluteCARE since these are the patients for whom aggressive, intensive attention might be most valuable, both in improving health and in decreasing total costs of care. However, they also have sites that take relatively healthy individuals, such as one at Dartmouth for employees.

An example is their program in Atlantic City, New Jersey, developed by Dr. Fernandopulle before establishing Iora Health but based on the same principles. Patients were given incentives through waived co-payments and pharmaceuticals to join. For every 1,200 patients, there is a team of two PCPs, an NP, six health coaches, two administrative staff, and a part-time nutritionist, psychologist and social worker. Initially, it was a partnership between a large multi-employer trust fund for service workers and a not-for-profit health system but later opened to other payers such as Horizon Blue Cross. They use a team-based approach and a proactive care system based on a registry of queries and event triggers. Within one year, based on a nationally-validated survey created by the Agency for Healthcare Research and Quality (AHRQ), there was a strong improvement in basics such as access to care, time and respect, communication with the patient and care coordination. Blood pressure and diabetes control improved, and smoking rates declined from 21 to 11 percent for a quit rate of a remarkable 48 percent. Days that were not productive at work dropped from an average of 17 to 9 days per year. Total costs of care decreased by 12 percent, driven by large decreases in hospital admissions (41 percent), ER visits (48 percent) and outpatient procedures (23 percent).

MedLion

MedLion was founded by husband and wife team Samir and Hisana Qamar, both family physicians. The MedLion concept is to assist PCPs converting to direct primary care either completely or in stages. They have over 200 PCPs on the rolls as of fall, 2014 and are growing rapidly. MedLion offers physicians the legal, administrative and other advantages of an organization so that during the conversion the PCP avoids the pitfalls of insurance commissioner wrath, patient anger at "abandonment," etc. The PCP remains independent but contracts with MedLion for these and other functions. MedLion CEO Dr. Samir Qamar believes that the populace is not yet ready for a mass conversion to direct primary care. One major reason is that most individuals just do not understand what "high impact" primary care can offer in the way of better care, less expensive care, avoidance of the need for specialists and more attention to wellness and prevention of illness.

On the other hand, he finds that employers, anxious from continuously rising healthcare expenses are amenable to innovative approaches to better care that reduce their total costs. MedLion offers the employer – their smallest has three employees and the largest has over 100,000 – a membership plan for about $50 per month per employee plus a $10 visit payment. There are no exclusions for preexisting conditions, age, full or part time status. Not only employees but family members can join. MedLion will connect the employer with an insurer that offers a high deductible catastrophic policy to complement the primary care. Generally the employer pays the membership fee each month and may or may not pay for the visit fee. Many employers will place a sum into an HSA account for the employee to use, including for the visit fees. Total costs for the employer (and for the employees' share of the now less expensive insurance premium) decline immediately compared to what it was paying previously for comprehensive insurance. And as time proceeds, the total costs decline further as the employees' health improves and productivity expands allowing the cost of the catastrophic insurance element to be further reduced.

Dr. Qamar argues that states will begin to appreciate the value of direct primary care for their employees just as do large and small companies since state governments carry a large healthcare obligation and, just like private enterprise employers, their costs are rising rapidly. What about Medicare and Medicaid? He anticipates that there will be continued pilot programs within Medicare Advantage that over time will demonstrate the value of this approach. The question for Medicaid administrators to overcome is not that high impact primary care costs more which of course it does compared to today's standard primary care. Rather they need to recognize that the total costs of care are reduced and quite dramatically while quality and satisfaction go up. Once they stop focusing on the cost of primary care and instead focus on total costs, perhaps they will appreciate the value of comprehensive primary care.

It Is all About Innovation

Change is coming to primary care, and the innovators and entrepreneurs are often those with a stake in the outcome. Primary Care Progress is developing advocacy, educating at the grassroots level to gain popular support for change and for excellence in primary care. Casey Health Institute is committed to an integrative model that connects a team-based model of primary care with complementary disciplines and a strong wellness component. AbsoluteCARE places added resources at the disposal of the team to offer superior care to those who might be termed the "sickest of the sick." Iora Health likewise uses added resources such as limited patients per PCP or NP, and the use of health coaches, nutritionists, and social workers. MedLion (next chapter) assists PCPs to convert to direct primary care and concurrently works with employers to offer a combined DPC approach to their employees coupled with a high deductible catastrophic ("true") insurance policy.

The message is clear: It costs more for this style of primary care, but the results in quality and total costs are striking.

CHAPTER SEVENTEEN

INNOVATORS: EMPLOYERS WHO GOT IT RIGHT

John Torinus, Jr., board chair and former CEO of Serigraph, Inc., understands the value of taking care of his employees. "Helping employees improve their health is right for the company's bottom line and is doing right by our employees. Healthier employees are happier, demonstrate less absenteeism ... and are more productive. This is a win for everyone involved."

CEOs must make healthcare a strategic priority since it is one of the top three costs for any company. Healthcare costs can make the company non-competitive if not managed well. However, making this a strategic priority means being proactive and involved – not just providing insurance. It is not just a cost issue for the HR department to solve, it is a strategic issue aimed at keeping employees well.

When more than 100 industry CEOs met for a Wall Street Journal conference to discuss the most pressing issues, they agreed to five top overall priorities, one which was healthcare.[94] Their recommendations included having "government and industry seek better healthcare outcomes," finding agreement on how to measure quality in care, when to use evidence-based approaches, eliminating waste including unnecessary services and administrative inefficiencies, and achieving price transparency. I believe that each of these can be met by addressing the crisis in primary care according to recommendations presented in this book.

Employers have seen their healthcare costs increase dramatically over the years. To compensate, they have passed at least part of that cost to employees in various ways, requiring them to pay for an increased portion of the premium, significant co-pays with each physician visit, and policies that restrict individuals to a narrow network of doctors and hospitals. This approach has not worked to slow the inexorable rise of medical care costs because it attacks the wrong problem. Instead, companies must institute approaches to improve health and maintain wellness of the employee (and those employees' families) and to assure that employees (and their families) receive outstanding primary care, including proactive population-style healthcare. To make this work, it is critical for employees to have a stake in the financial transactions that transpire. They need to be an engaged consumer of medical care. The combination will reduce costs considerably. Here are some approaches that progressive companies are following.

Company Wellness Plans

Large companies such as General Mills and Safeway have demonstrated the utility of wellness programs. Employees are invited to voluntarily participate in company-sponsored programs that are designed for behavior modification, such as nutrition, fitness, chronic stress reduction and smoking cessation. The employees (and sometimes the employee' family members) who participate are rewarded with a reduction in their share of the health care premium. Given that employers are continually increasing employee share, this reduction can be a real benefit to a person's paycheck. Large corporations often create these programs in-house, but both small and large businesses turn to wellness companies to create a turnkey approach for a single larger company or a group of smaller companies in a defined geographic region. Workplace wellness programs should improve employee health, but until now, there was no definitive proof. New evidence shows an opt-in program with biometric testing and a personal wellness profile to guide individualized health coaching, combined with financial incentives, led to improved health parameters, improved health age and reduced healthcare costs.[95]

Here are some of the specific findings: Compared to nonparticipants, the participant's claims increased at a lower rate, and there were fewer claims per person. For those with elevated blood pressure, the average systolic pressure was 170 mmHg, which was reduced by 34 over the three-year study. For diastolic, the average of 105 was reduced by 18 mmHg. For those with elevated glucose, the starting average was 164.4 and dropped by 31 over the three years. Those at the greatest risk for cancer improved their lifestyle score by nearly 32 points, or 41 percent.

According to my interview with Darrell Moon, CEO of Orriant, a wellness company, there are a few key ingredients that make for a successful wellness program. The majority of employees (and spouses) need to work one-on-one with a health coach to develop a self-directed plan for behavioral improvement. Individual care and concern by the health coach is the most effective intervention. Employees need to like their coach, which I further interpret to mean they trust their coach. Individual accountability must be an integral part of the program. The focus should be on those with health risks, which most Americans have. Getting the men in the company involved is important – women are more likely to volunteer early, so there has to be extra effort to attract the men.

Major health risks from lifestyle factors include being overweight (two-thirds of the American population), lack of adequate exercise (probably more than half of Americans), chronic stress (almost everyone) and smoking (still about 20 percent of the population). High blood pressure can also be lifestyle directed. These five factors in turn lead to chronic illnesses such as heart disease, stroke, chronic lung and kidney disease – the diseases that account for 75-85 percent of all claims paid by healthcare insurance.

The cost of wellness programs, whether done in-house or with a consultant, can be self-funding, which means those who opt in get lower premiums and those who do not have higher premiums. But the more valuable benefits accrue to both the employer and employee. Staff become healthier, and healthier employees use fewer total healthcare resources. This lowers company insurance costs or slows the growth of premiums, often dramatically. The employees benefit from better health, will likely be more productive, have fewer absentee days and have greater job satisfaction. That is a win-win for employee and employer alike.

Company-based Primary Care Programs

Patients need doctors who take time to listen. Employers need programs that reduce costs and improve the health of their staff. These sometimes disparate needs can come together in a new model for effective primary healthcare.

Some employers are turning to firms such as QuadMed to initiate care models that address both requirements. Transitioning from being a purchaser of health insurance to an investor in employee health and productivity is a significant change for most companies. QuadMed started when Harry Quadracci, founder and CEO of parent company QuadGraphics, decided to work on improving his employees' health rather than only provide care when they got sick. QuadMed began as a wellness program and evolved into enhanced primary care. For their 6,800 employees in Wisconsin, there are three on-site clinics. Each includes PCPs, nurses and other providers and a pharmacy, laboratory, radiology suite and other key resources such as nutritionists. These resources allow for close care and monitoring of patients with complex chronic illnesses. There are multiple other clinics for the remaining approximately 13,000 employees in other states where QuadGraphics has plants. Some of these are not large enough to justify an in-house pharmacy or radiology suite. Over time QuadMed began to sell this approach to other companies, making modifications as necessary for the specific needs of the company. The employer is generally self-insured, has a large enough employee base to justify the clinic resources, is committed to employee health and wellness, and wants to reduce its total costs of health care. Although the employer has no access to patient records or visits, it is important for the employer to set up communication to encourage use of the clinic, including incentives built into the health insurance plan.

Under the program, a full-service primary care clinic is funded by the company at or near the employer's site of business. Employees are welcome, but not required, to participate at no cost or a small fee of about $10 per visit. Some employers make the clinics available to family members as well. Each individual is assigned a primary care physician who is paid by salary, not fee-for-service. Given the shortage of PCPs, a growing number of nurse practitioners or physician assistants under PCP supervision are being employed with good success and acceptance. The PCP completes a full initial evaluation that lasts 60 minutes or more and then sees the individual as often as necessary for as long as necessary. The expectation is that the patient and doctor will develop a long-term trusting relationship. Individuals can schedule appointments often on the same or next day, and there is extensive use of mobile technologies, an electronic medical record, telemedicine and other advanced techniques. For individuals with a chronic illness, the clinic nurses work with the PCP to coordinate care, and the PCP communicates directly with any specialist before referring and after the visit.

QuadMed provides, at an additional cost, a trained and certified nurse educator to work with employees who have diabetes, hypertension or asthma. If the numbers are not sufficient to justify a full-time person, the interactions can be done "face to face" via teleconferencing between patient and nurse. These nurses can be available for employees who have not opted to use the clinic for their primary care. The employer creates certain incentives for enrolling with the nurse educator, such as offering medications for the condition with no co-pays. The nurses tend to work primarily with the highest risk individuals and refer those with less serious issues to the nutritionist or health coach for general wellness programs.

The clinic manages wellness and preventive programs with health coaching and lifestyle behavior management. This might include nutrition counseling, fitness counseling, stress management and smoking cessation. If the company has a wellness program with another provider, QuadMed partners with that provider to create seamless programs. It is an employer wellness program and a primary care program rolled into one. It is population health to the extent that the PCP and the team proactively interact with each participant rather than wait for an employee or patient to call or visit with a problem.

QuadMed and the employer agree to a set of performance measures, including utilization/penetration of the clinic (Are employees actually using it?), patient satisfaction (Do they like what they get?), quality outcomes (standard measures used nationally such as blood pressure control, diabetic control, and up-to-date immunizations), adherence to the budget, and a return on the employer's investment at a pre-agreed level.

Some companies that would like this model are not large enough to justify the expense, but they can partner with other nearby businesses for a shared clinic. Alternatively, a clinic can be established that is not "full service" but uses extensive telemedicine and other technologies to connect the patient with various providers not on site.

QuadMed calls this approach "on-site" primary care in a holistic, patient-centered model with convenient access and the development of a strong provider-patient relationship. The aim is to completely avoid the "production model" so often found today in primary care. As Harry Quadracci stated, "We'll keep you well; and by the way, if you get sick, we'll take care of that, too."[96]

I had the opportunity to interview a patient/employee who uses a QuadMed primary care clinic for herself and her family. She told me that she previously used an HMO and that the maximum time per visit was 15 minutes. "I needed to be sure I had my questions ready and that I did not forget to ask anything in the limited amount of time. Often, we didn't even get to cover everything. Now I use the QuadMed clinic and it is completely different. I once asked my doctor, 'How is it that you have so much time to spend with me?' She responded, 'You needed it today. That is what I am here for.' I also feel like the clinic addresses my health issues before they become serious, costly problems. Recently, I had an appointment scheduled and the doctor called me personally to say that she needed to reschedule. I could not believe that she called herself. When I didn't reschedule right away, a nurse followed up to be sure I had a new appointment.

"My husband uses the clinic as well. As a pre-diabetic, his doctor has been able to guide him in making meaningful lifestyle changes to bring down his sugar levels. At first, he needed to be on medication but eventually he was able to stop taking those medications altogether. He is healthier as a result, leading a much more active, happy life. As a big bonus, we are saving on the cost of the medications. The care we both get is so much better than any of us were getting before."

Another firm, WeCare TLC, calls their similar model "medical risk management," a term generally thought of in medicine as programs and policies to reduce the potential for malpractice claims. Used here, however, it has a completely different meaning. The concept is called medical risk management because the driving principle is identification and management of ongoing medical problems while at the same time addressing potential health risks for the future. It is a company-wide approach to population health management. It is taken from the concept of enterprise risk management, which seeks to identify and mitigate corporate risk as a strategic advantage.[97] It includes management of risk not just from a downside perspective but from an upside or positive perspective as well. This is another example of the employer thinking about health risk management from this strategic perspective, not only as a tactical cost avoidance effort.

In these models of primary care, the employer fully pays for the primary care services, so there can be a significant savings for the employee (patient) and family members. The employee receives quality healthcare with a strong emphasis on maintaining wellness, active prevention, early detection of chronic illnesses and care coordination. The result is a healthier workforce, which should lead to greater productivity, greater workforce satisfaction and reduced health insurance cost increases for both employers and employees.

In discussing WeCare with Brian Klepper, a principal and chief development officer, he observed that innovators are creating new improved methods to manage care while avoiding "rampant" waste. He feels that most are mission driven leading to a sense of real purpose. Among their principle characteristics are business models that create real value for clients/employees/patients; the models are full continuum and inter-disciplinary; the basis is comprehensive primary care but with control over downstream care; accepting financial risk; and the potential to grow rapidly because success is rewarded with scale. Among the companies or organizations discussed in this book, he mentioned Iora Health, Qliance and of course WeCare as fitting his six characteristics.

Whatever terminology used, the most frequent underlying motivator for the employer is to save company resources, improve health and wellness, and provide quality care management. When done appropriately, it has beneficial health effects for the individual (and family), saves the employee substantial money and offers better health all around. Definitely a triple win.

Critical to success – and that triple win – is a contract between PCP (or PCP group) with the employer that allows the physician the time needed for close listening, thinking, coordinating chronic care and quality preventive care, an appropriately limited number of patients/employees (and family members). Trying to cut corners with high PCP/NP throughput will only negate the opportunities for quality benefit and total cost reductions. That approach is a waste of valuable employer resources and will not improve health, save money or improve productivity of the workforce.

These types of employer-sponsored primary care programs should not be equated with urgent care or episodic care clinics within or near a company.

These are usually designed to accommodate the minor issues that crop up among employees such as a sprain, urinary tract infection, or strep throat. These clinics are certainly valuable and helpful, but they are definitely not the same as an enhanced primary care model that seeks to develop a long-term relationship between doctor and patient.

Insurer or Company-Sponsored Membership Style Primary Care

Another variant is appearing for smaller businesses. Rather than establish their own primary care clinic, these companies have chosen to purchase the retainer/membership for their employees in a direct primary care practice. Alternatively, they place a sum of money in the employee's HSA that can be used to pay the membership fee for the DPC physician of the employee's choice. Although the dollars come from an employer, they are managed by the employee, which means more personal accountability.

At least one insurer has decided to partner with a direct primary care (retainer/membership type) practice. The Nevada Health Co-op, an insurer on the Nevada health exchange, offers policies with Turntable Heath, a membership-based primary care provider. A person can select the Co-op in the exchange and purchase a policy that combines a membership with Turntable along with a catastrophic policy with a high deductible. The Co-op pays an $80 monthly fee to Turntable from the premiums collected. Turntable combines a PCP and a health coach for each patient, includes classes on health and wellness, and otherwise functions like other membership primary care practices.

MedLion

MedLion, described in the previous chapter, is a Nevada-based company that offers a membership style primary care practice in 15 locations with aspirations to go nationwide. It charges $59 per month plus a $10 visit charge. To date, about 75 percent of their patients derive from contracts with employer self-insurance plans. The founders believe that employers much more so than individuals or insurers are the first to recognize the value of expanded primary care both for the health of their employees and for controlling healthcare costs.

Iora Health

Iora Health, discussed in the previous chapter, largely deals directly with employers or unions who purchase complete expanded primary care for their employees or members. As with MedLion they believe that the place to start is with employers and some enlightened insurers or their sponsors such as union health trust funds.

Physician's Care Direct

Physician's Care Direct in North Carolina, mentioned in Chapter 14, offers self-insured employers a package of direct primary care, along with insurance for specialty care and hospitalization. The employer pays Physician's Care Direct, which in turn pays for DPC for expanded primary care with episodic care, common labs, radiology, vaccines, extensive preventive care and chronic disease management. There are no co-pays or deductibles. Specialty care and hospitalization is covered by the insurance component and may include co-pays and deductibles as determined by the employer. The concept is to convert a completely fixed "insurance" cost to a much smaller fixed cost for catastrophic care and leave the rest variable for primary care. The aim is to improve health and wellness with first-rate primary care, thus reducing that variable cost substantially.

Healthcare as a Business Strategy

Throughout this book, I have written primarily from the perspective of what primary care physicians can do to not only improve the health of their patients while reducing total costs of care yet also reclaim their right to practice in a non-frustrating environment with a limited numbers of patient visits per day. John Torinus of Serigraph, mentioned at the beginning of this chapter, approaches improving healthcare from the perspective of a business leader faced with rising health care costs.

He notes that CEOs need to think about the long term for their companies and for their employees. The company and the employee together spend about $16,000 per year per family for insurance today. An employee who works for a company for 25-40 years represents an insurance expenditure over a lifetime career that could be as much as $400,000 to $640,000 in today's dollars. This drives home the point that it makes sense to have a long-term view of employee health, beginning with an aggressive approach to maintain wellness, actively reduce risk factors and manage disease as it occurs. A population health approach.

Torinus observes that the current health care system focuses on specialty care though it needs to focus on the care recipient with high quality primary care. But to be effective, the patient/consumer/employee must be engaged. The current healthcare system disengages the patient – it removes responsibility because the patient is not the customer of the doctor.

In his company, expenses were rising to double digits by 2003, but with their new plan in place, it dropped to 2 percent or less per year continuously for more than a decade.

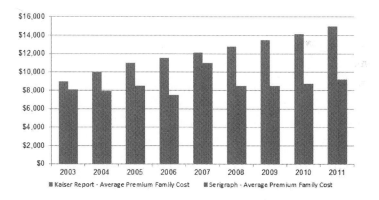

Torinus' "prescription" for all companies – and what his company initiated beginning in 2004 – follows: First, every company, including small companies, should self-insure with an added stop-loss catastrophic policy. Second, employees should be offered only a consumer-directed healthcare policy (CDHP), in essence a high-deductible plan (often about $2,500) with either an associated health savings account (HSA) or a health related account (HRA). The company should prefund the account with an amount (often about $1,500) that the individual can use for any health care needs with the assumption that he or she will spend it more wisely. This encourages employee/patient engagement. Third, the company should insist that each provider have price transparency. Since that is often difficult to obtain, Serigraph uses various companies such as Alithias Inc. to provide that for them to compare providers. For example, they determine the all-inclusive price (gastroenterologist, anesthesiologist and facility fee), along with quality data of colonoscopies, at the nearest five centers and then rank them. The employee or family member who needs the colonoscopy is told that, for example, the company sees it as appropriate preventive care and will cover the cost, in this case up to $1,500. This amount will pay fully for four of the five local centers, but if he or she selects a provider that charges more, they are on the hook for the remainder.

Fourth, if the company is large enough, it should provide an on-site primary care clinic at no cost to the individual. At Serigraph, the clinic includes a concierge-type physician, meaning that the physician is salaried, has a low number of patients under care and gives extensive time and energy to each employee/family member patient. The clinic also includes a nurse practitioner, health coach, dietician and chiropractor. If the company is too small to justify a full-fledged clinic, then the company can pay the retainer for a nearby direct primary care/membership/concierge physician who works with others, such as the health coach. Fifth, the clinic, with special attention by the health coach, gives all employees a health risk assessment annually and then works one-on-one with each employee (and family member) at no cost to maintain wellness and health, including the use of behavioral change programs around diet, nutrition, exercise, stress management and smoking cessation. Sixth, there is intense management of chronic diseases by the clinic staff and coordination of specialist visits when needed. Seventh, Serigraph uses what Torinus calls "Centers of Value" for procedures beyond those done by the primary care physician. These are doctors or institutions that have outstanding quality records yet a competitive price for, say, a knee replacement. Serigraph gives their employees $2,000 toward the deductible or totally covers the deductible for the surgery when they make use of these Centers of Value. Eighth, his company gives generic drugs for free, and all of the above prevention and wellness programs are supplied free of charge.

Finally, the company provides free counseling for developing advanced directives and, in the event that an individual requires end-of-life care, hospice is available free of charge.

I notice that his company spends considerably on extensive and comprehensive primary care, including wellness maintenance, proactive prevention and chronic care management, but it is rewarded in return with lower total costs and healthier workers.

These approaches are based on fundamental principles, including individual responsibility, marketplace discipline (installing consumerism and steering specialty care to the best quality and price), proactive care (maintaining employees' health and wellness and giving extensive care to those with chronic illnesses), and sound management (putting those who pay, including the employer and the employee, in charge).

Torinus suggests there are multiple rewards for following this basic approach. I added the second sentence since he implied it but did not write it.

1) The reward for business is a healthier workforce and more affordable healthcare expenditures.
2) The reward for individuals is more health and wellness, less illness and fewer dollars spent.
3) The reward for high value providers is more business.
4) The reward for entrepreneurs comes if they innovate with better care provided at lower cost
5) There *could be* a reward for taxpayers - if government (federal, state and local) used these approaches.[98]

As employers (and insurers) recognize that high quality expanded primary care may cost more upfront but actually reduces their total costs and increases employee productivity, I predict that they will increasingly gravitate to these types of plans. This is the concept of making employee health a company strategic priority rather than just seeing health insurance as a cost management concern.

CHAPTER EIGHTEEN

RETAIL PRIMARY CARE: READILY AVAILABLE AND INEXPENSIVE BUT NOT RELATIONSHIP CARE

With primary care in turmoil, shortages of PCPs, lack of ready access for many patients and high costs, many corporations are sensing a potential profit from primary care. AbsoluteCARE, Iora Health, MedLion, QuadMed and WeCare LLC are examples already discussed. Here are a few more.

Large Medical Group Corporations

DaVita, a national provider of dialysis services for those with chronic kidney failure, has acquired HealthCare Partners, a company that manages and operates large medical groups and affiliated physician networks in multiple states with nearly 800,000 patients in managed care programs. They also have a subsidiary called Paladina Health (the name was chosen because paladin means a defender or advocate of a noble cause) that helps self-insured employers to manage their primary care. Their model uses independent primary care physicians that are assigned a panel of employer's staff and operates as a medical home with 24/7 access to the PCP, wellness coaching, same or next-day appointments, and proactive physician outreach. Presumably, they do all of this only by reducing the physician's total patients under care. Their web site argues that Paladina can reduce the employer's total costs by 12 percent net of Paladina's fee, often with a reduction closer to 20-30 percent.

In another effort, HealthCare Partners has linked with Independence Blue Cross to jointly create an entity called Tandigm Health. Tandigm seeks to engage a large group of PCPs to care for a segment of Independence's insured members. The plan is to create incentives for the PCPs to improve primary care quality rather than quantity, and in the process, lower the total costs of care. The initial service area is southeast Philadelphia, which today has one of the highest rates of hospitalization and total expenses. Tandigm offers new analytical tools to the PCPs, provides training in complex chronic illness care coordination to the PCP and offers increased access to added services such as home care, especially for the frail and elderly.

Urgent Care Clinics

Urgent care companies began to proliferate 30 years ago but have gained traction in recent years as emergency room wait times rapidly lengthened. Urgent care is less expensive than the ER, is open 24/7 or at least begins early and continues late, and the staff is dedicated to minor medical problems that need rapid or immediate attention. Urgent care centers do not require an appointment like a doctor's office but most encourage a pre-call or an online connection to set a definitive time for the visit; meaning little or no waiting time. Unlike the clinics in the chain pharmacies discussed below, these urgent care centers are usually equipped to handle broken bones, minor surgery and laceration stitching. Most urgent care centers have a physician on site most of the time and available by phone at all times. Costs vary by type of treatment, but an average bill might be about $100-$140 (not unlike the cost of visiting a PCP) compared to more than $500-$1,000 for an emergency room visit for the same problem. Typical co-pays for those with insurance might be about $40 versus $200 for the same problem seen in the ER. Prices are posted for all to see so there is cost transparency. Insurance is accepted, yet it is also a venue that appeals to those with a high-deductible insurance policy.

Urgent care centers often become de facto primary care physicians for many individuals who do not have insurance or simply cannot easily access a primary care provider. Although they do not provide long term relationship medicine, many smaller centers with just a few providers on staff can and do offer a more personalized service.

As a general rule, these are not centers that cater to dealing with chronic illnesses like heart failure, diabetes or chronic lung disease. That said, the patient with recurrent asthmatic attacks might well use the urgent care center rather than an ER and so too might the patient with brittle diabetes or an exacerbation of heart failure.

For some of the same reasons, urgent care centers are generally not focused on the geriatric population with its many chronic illnesses. Yet, these are individuals that are often in greatest need of rapid attention, attention that could prevent an ER visit or even a hospitalization. Many nursing home patients get sent to the ER late at night when the nursing home staff encounters a problem such as fever, dehydration, breathing difficulties, etc. A relationship with an urgent care center, ideally using telemedicine technology, could result in many fewer hospitalizations and ER visits, better care and less physical and emotional trauma to the elderly resident.

Another innovation is to pair a subscription primary care model with an urgent care center. Conceptually, a person, an insurer or an employer purchases the subscription, which offers the individual unlimited access to the urgent care center with an expanded primary care program. For example, EveraHealth partners with urgent care chains and charges $40-$50 per month, or $480-$600 per year, for unlimited primary care. Their plan uses the direct primary care concept of decoupling the doctor from the insurer and eliminates the requirements of coding, billing and preauthorizations. Since the care takes place at an urgent care center, the added capital requirements for the primary care program are minimal. The individual is welcome to make an appointment with the primary care provider at the center or show up on an urgent basis with no added charge.

The concept, still to be proven in practice, as described by chairman and CEO Robert Enslein, is to "not only take advantage of underutilized capacity in the clinics, but also drive down the overall cost of care on a long term basis. By improving the cash flow characteristics of the clinics through this subscription based model, the urgent care clinics can better model for growth, improvement in care, and expansion of services."

Although this model probably does not mean true relationship-based care with a strong bind between an individual doctor and individual patient, it provides episodic care, urgent care, an annual exam, preventive services and other elements of primary care. When the physician (or nurse practitioner) is not available, the clinic is still open extended hours for urgent issues. The business model assumes that the PCP salary and overheads can be covered with about 10-12 patient visits per day, substantially less than is typical in a PCP private office so visits can be as long as needed. Added benefits can be discounted laboratory testing and medications available at wholesale prices.

Primary Care Clinics within Retail Stores

Walgreens and CVS pharmacy chains are aggressively developing primary care venues within their stores. Although many people may scoff at retailers like Walgreens or CVS entering this arena, they have the potential to reach people who may not otherwise be able to get the medical care they need. For some years their pharmacists have offered immunizations, especially flu, shingles and pneumonia vaccines. Many are expanding this offering. The pharmacist is being used more than previously for patient advice, drug compliance monitoring, and appropriate dosing (such as Coumadin for atrial fibrillation.) In addition, Walgreens and CVS have created retail primary care centers within the walls of some of their pharmacy superstores. Their approaches are somewhat different although the underlying strategy is the same for both. The idea is to deliver episodic care to those in need with a motto of, essentially, "You're sick, we're quick." Originally initiated by James D'Orta, MD, an entrepreneur and emergency medicine physician, and sold to CVS, it is known as MinuteClinic with 800 units nationwide and an expectation to grow to at least 1,500. The CVS health services are staffed primarily by nurse practitioners or physician assistants. CVS has relationships with physicians available to offer advice to the NP or PA on request. Counseling for nutrition, weight loss and smoking cessation are commonplace as well. About 85 percent of clients have insurance and most of those have their own primary care physician.

Later, Dr. D'Orta and others worked with Duane Reade, a large pharmacy chain in New York City. Duane Reade partnered with Consumer Health Services of Washington, D.C., to open primary care clinics in some of their stores staffed with physicians. Called "Dr. Walk-In Medical Care" or sometimes "Doctor on Premises," they found it successful as a product offering because it brought customers into their stores, which generated downstream sales of drugs and other products. Customers tend to be those who might have their own PCP but do not want to wait days to see the doctor for a minor but troubling issue.

They find that the cost is low, the wait is short and the doctor is well-trained. Dr. Walk-In conducts exams, basic treatment services, health screenings and vaccinations. It is physician-centric rather than focused on nurse practitioners. The physician offers episodic and semi-urgent care but does not invest in a PCP-patient long-term relationship. Rather, he or she offers a referral back to your PCP or to a specialist if indicated. The clinics were highly successful and when Duane Reade was acquired by Walgreens, Walgreens decided to purchase the clinics from the founders and expand the concept nationally as Healthcare Clinic, with a switch from physician providers to nurse practitioners.

The Affordable Care Act is one driver of this expansion of retail sites. With more people on Medicaid or subsidized insurance, the need for primary care is expanding at a time when there are too few primary care providers. More health policies, including those through the insurance exchanges, come with high deductibles so the patient must pay the primary care provider. The retail clinic is sometimes less expensive than a fee-for-service doctor visit. Another factor is convenience. These retail clinics tend to be open early in the morning, late in the evening, on weekends and without appointments. Prices are posted for all to see so there is cost transparency. Insurance is accepted, yet it is also a venue that appeals to those with a high-deductible insurance policy. The venue helps those with a PCP who is at a distance or cannot be accessed immediately and those who need treatment without losing time from work or school. The term "episodic primary care" seems appropriate because the provider is not representing himself or herself as a personal, long-time primary care provider, but rather as a provider who is readily available for pressing issues, such as a urinary tract infection, a minor injury, immunizations and counseling. This model is "family medical care made easy," Walgreens says.

Walgreens partnered with a new developing company called Theranos to provide on-site blood testing using Theranos technology, which uses a few drops of blood to test for more than 200 components. Results are available in a few hours, posted online and sent to both patient and PCP. This adds to the convenience factor and may draw people away from commercial laboratories.

Target has recently announced that it is opening primary care clinics in many of its stores beginning in California with an approach quite similar to CVS and Walgreens except that they have partnered with Kaiser Permanente to staff the clinics with NPs plus physician telemedicine backup.

Duane Reade, Walgreens, Target and CVS clearly understand that if they can leverage the healthcare marketplace to have a real stake in primary care delivery, then they will benefit from the downstream revenue of primary care. If you are in the store, you will also buy your drugs, supplements and other health and non-health products there. For many individuals, this is the entry point into the healthcare system. In some ways, this is unfortunate since primary care, as we have seen, is not solely about "episodic care." Comprehensive primary care, which the CVS and Walgreens clinics do not provide, is about long-term relationship medicine with intensive preventive care, maintenance of health and wellness, early action on risk factors, attention to those with chronic illnesses, coordination of specialists when needed and occasional episodic care of minor issues. That said, Walgreens and CVS offer a much-needed and appreciated venue for rapid access and care when a PCP is not otherwise available due to shortages, distance, or time constraints. And it is inexpensive.

Walmart, America's largest retailer with as many pharmacies as the chains, will soon begin primary clinics as well, beginning with a few stores and using QuadMed (see previous chapter) as the vendor. Unlike healthcare organizations that currently rent space from Walmart for their operations, Walmart's Care Clinic will be more like a full-service primary care service staffed by nurse practitioners with PCP backup. Their employees will pay only $4 per visit, and customers will pay $40 per encounter. The plan is to be open for 12 hours on weekdays and 8 hours on weekends. The Walmart Care Clinic will offer care for selected chronic conditions such as mild anxiety, asthma, uncomplicated diabetes, high blood pressure and elevated cholesterol, osteoarthritis and osteoporosis. When the requirements are beyond the scope of the nurse practitioner, the patient will be referred to an appropriate specialist. Each clinic will have the capacity for basic laboratory testing such as blood glucose, blood counts, rapid strep throat test, urinalysis, and pregnancy testing. Vaccines such as influenza, shingles, pneumonia, hepatitis A and B, chickenpox and HPV will be available. With an arrangement with Quest Laboratories, the clinic can draw bloods or obtain other samples to send for most other testing needs, sparing the patient the need to go to a separate facility. After test runs, we can expect Walmart, a disruptive innovator, to aggressively clone their clinics nationwide. Will Walmart become the country's largest purveyor of primary care, just as it has for food and toys? More importantly, will Walmart appreciate the importance of an appropriate patient-to-provider number to bolster real relationship medicine?

Many physicians disparage the creation of these types of primary care venues. Their logic, not unreasonable, is that individuals will do better with a PCP who offers comprehensive care. Their argument is correct except that it is hard for many to find such a physician, and even if they do, the PCP may not be available in off hours. Utilizing an urgent care clinic or a clinic at Walgreens, CVS or Walmart is certainly better than going to the busy ER for a minor issue, both in cost and time. These sites may also prove a better venue for getting blood drawn for testing and rapidly getting the information back to the PCP. Rather than complaining, perhaps a better approach is for PCPs to find ways to partner with these clinics. Partnerships, not turf battles, will be key for the future.

House Calls on Demand

A few enterprising groups (such as House Call Doctor Los Angeles and Medicast) arrange for a PCP to make a prompt house call on the spot by credit card. The overheads are low with no nurse, receptionist or office. Patients summon the doctor via telephone or an app similar to those for taxi or Uber limousine service. An on-call doctor in the area arrives at your home (or hotel room for a traveler) within two hours to give you personalized attention. The charge is $200 to $400. It may sound expensive, but the concept is that it costs much less than the $1,000 it would cost at the ER, and you do not have to hang around the ER waiting room. For those with a high-deductible policy but no PCP – or at least not one who is readily available – this is definitely cheaper. It is more expensive than one of the retail clinics at the drug store chains or most urgent care centers, but you receive prompt care without leaving home (or hotel room.) It is not long-term relationship-based primary care but it is efficient when you need help.

Concierge Medicine House-Call Based

Some physicians have decided to limit their practice to house calls only and do so with a direct primary care model. For example, Marc Tanenbaum, MD speaks of himself as North Atlanta's first concierge pediatrician but limits his practice to house calls only. After more than 25 years in a regular practice, he converted to direct primary care. He has a receptionist reachable by phone or email but he has no public office. Rather, he cares for his patients only in their home. He charges a modest retainer once per quarter and a fee for each visit, the latter to discourage home visits that could as well be dealt with over the phone. Most patients can be seen the same day and as with other DPC-style practices, he gives his patients' parents his cell phone number and will respond at any time. With no office, no insurance billing and only a receptionist, his practice expenses are very low. He finds that there are two drawbacks for his patients (parents). The first is that many insurance companies will not pay for childhood vaccinations that he administers because he is "out of network." Since an infant's immunizations during the first 18 months of life can add up to nearly $2000 this becomes an impediment for the parents. The second issue relates to the home visit fee. He offers parents a form which they can send to the insurer for reimbursement of his home visits. In this way, even if the parents have a high deductible policy, the visit fee goes against the deductible. The problem is that now the parents learn just how often insurers deny claims or request further information, a problem not appreciated when the typical fee-for-service doctor's office handles the billing; this obviously creates frustration among his parents. To overcome this, he will have his bookkeeper submit the billing (and deal with denials, etc.) for an added $10 fee per visit.

House-call only physicians do not all operate in a DPC or concierge manner and to date they are not a common practice option but there are associations that assist doctors convert their practices and to assist patients find such physicians. Elderly patients especially may benefit from a house call style practice particularly when they cannot easily travel to the doctor's office.

Virtual Doctor Visits

If it is possible to provide episodic primary care at a pharmacy, at Wal-Mart, via home visits, etc., then why not do it via telemedicine or other electronic interconnection between patient and doctor? The advantage is that the individual can consult with a doctor at any time of day or night, not leave home or office and hopefully receive quality advice and treatment.

Among companies offering this "E-visit" service are MDLIVE, Teladoc, American Well and Doctor on Demand. Although each is different, all require you to register online and create a database with your health history and current medications. You then briefly describe your medical issue and request a consultation. You will be called or contacted by Skype within a few minutes or messaged online by a physician or nurse practitioner. These services are designed for straight-forward, non-emergent common problems, including minor infections, inflammation, minor sports injuries, sprains, and low back pain. The doctor will give advice and call your pharmacy with a prescription if needed. Some offer limited mental health assistance as well. Costs vary by company but fees for a single consultation are in the range of $30-$40 for most "visits" and $80-$100 for a mental health therapist, payable upfront by credit card.

Like the primary care services in the chain pharmacies, these offer episodic care but are not full-service primary care. Nevertheless, given that it is often difficult in today's environment to get an early appointment with your PCP or an appointment outside of business hours, these services will likely continue to proliferate. Plus, the expense and wait time are trivial compared to the ER.

Urgent Care, Walk in Clinics, and Emergency Care vs Direct Primary Care

Dr. Josh Umbehr, the founder at AtlasMD discussed in Chapter 14, offered an interesting opinion piece, titled "A solution to ER Overcrowding: Direct Care." He moonlights in a local ER and comments that about 80 percent of what he sees he could have treated in his primary care office at a lower cost. He states that he is required by hospital protocol to do multiple tests that he would not likely do in his own practice, which increase the costs of care to more than $500 per visit. Recognizing that they will often not be paid since the patient may not have insurance, about 50 percent of hospitals now charge a fee of about $150 in cash for those seeking care in the ER but not requiring true emergent help. Although the patient's insurance might pay for the ER visit, the patient is expected to pay the $150 fee. Further, for that same $150, Dr. Umbehr would not only treat the current issue but give a three-month membership to his practice. If the patient needed a follow-up, they would receive it at no extra cost, whereas an ER visit would be at least an additional $150 out of pocket.[99]

My thought: These can be valuable services when your PCP is not available and urgent care centers are critical (in place of the ER) when you need immediate care for a broken bone, series laceration or sudden severe asthma attack. But think back to the discussion of direct primary care in a membership model. The doctor gives you his or her cell phone to call 24/7 and will see you the same or next day. Membership plans are as low as $40 per month. It would be better to have a full-service PCP at your disposal through a membership or retainer approach than a doctor who does not know you, will not interact with you the next time you have an issue, and who can only deal with limited situations.

Concluding Thoughts on the Future

Primary care is rapidly transforming before our eyes. It is clear that the typical primary care private practice fee-for-service insurance reimbursement model is rapidly disappearing. It is being replaced with PCPs converting to direct primary care, PCPs working for hospitals, employer-sponsored primary care clinics, episodic care clinics such as at CVS and Walgreens, urgent care centers, E-visit and house call companies and now Walmart. Some of these approaches maintain the typical bond of trust between PCP and patient and offer expanded primary care. Others respond only to the episodic needs of the client, which can often be sufficient but cannot replace the relationship-based practice of the PCP who offers full service with a limited number of patients.

These are all responses to a problem that has been festering for decades, ever since insurance became available for primary care and insurers started limiting their expenses through price controls. This approach by insurers has been an unmitigated disaster that has not only backfired, but taken us backwards. We now have lower quality medical care at much higher rates than necessary. One result is that various corporations and organizations are trying to profit from the chaos in the primary care marketplace. Some will be useful and of high quality, but others will not. The positive message is that this is innovation, much needed as medical care delivery transforms.

Until we correct the primary care physician-to-patient ratio, this problem will continue to get worse. For the PCP who wishes to continue or start a private practice, direct primary care is one of the most promising options. The retainer or membership may be paid by the patient or employer. Perhaps even the insurers, including Medicare and Medicaid, will decide to transition to this approach since they can materially benefit from reduced total costs of the improved care. Alternatively, there are models that employ the PCP or pay a per-member per-month (PMPM) fee to the PCP at a rate that will reduce patient numbers and limit visits to a manageable number per day. Here again, employers may be at the forefront, followed slowly by insurers.

In each of the models of comprehensive primary care with fewer patients per PCP, patients will be the real beneficiaries as they will have access to care that will:

1. Maintain wellness and prevent chronic illnesses from occurring,
2. Provide appropriate prompt care of episodic needs, and
3. Provide thorough care for complex chronic illnesses, including coordination of the care among providers when needed.

It is about a return to relationship medicine combined with extensive wellness preservation, health maintenance and illness management. The result will be a healthier population and reduced healthcare costs.

For physicians still in a traditional private practice of primary care, there are a few options. They can stick with the status quo and hope that something may improve (not likely), join the local hospital and become employed (fewer administrative requirements but still productivity expectations and a loss of autonomy), look to a newly developing accountable care organization (valuable only if the payments to the PCP allow for fewer patients), look for an employer-based primary care clinic, or adapt with some form of direct pay model (fewer patients, same or possibly greater income, better care for your patients).

It is clear that the current reimbursement system for primary care cannot be sustained in the long term without modifications. It will collapse of its own weight and likely do so soon. Doctors who understand and agree that their role is to manage the vertical delivery of services – by offering extensive preventive care using a population health approach, managing the care of those with chronic illnesses, coordinating others involved in the care of chronic illness, and avoiding unnecessary referrals and testing – should expect to be rewarded.

In short, rather than tinkering with the current broken system, we should completely rework the way primary care is delivered and paid for to lead to much better care, much lower total costs and more satisfied patients and doctors.

Part V

FINDING A CURE

There are straightforward ways to ensure you receive the best possible healthcare. This section begins with recommendations from primary care physicians about what you can do to help your PCP (and other providers) care for you.

The next chapter spells out specifics of what primary care physicians, insurers, employers, elected officials, academic medical center leaders and especially you – the patient or potential patient – can do to change the paradigm to a more effective approach to primary care. Working together, we can create a *primary care system that offers high quality care to satisfied patients through enthusiastic and energized physicians at a reasonable price that lowers the total cost of care.*

Chapter Nineteen

GETTING THE BEST POSSIBLE HEALTHCARE

Robert is in his mid-40s, about 20 pounds overweight, and otherwise in good health. He began to have annoying pain in his mid-back. It seemed to be related to meals and often occurred after he went to bed, but it was inconsistent. After a month, he went to his PCP. The PCP was uncertain but suspected a possible gallstone. Gallstones can cause pain in the back, usually located near the scapula on the right side, but Robert's pain was more diffuse, lower and across the width of his back. The PCP, now at the end of his 15 minutes with Robert, sent him to a gastroenterologist, who took a brief history and ordered a battery of tests. The tests were all negative. The doctor next ordered a CT scan of his abdomen. There were no gallstones, but something about the scan was unusual. The radiologist report indicated that he could not rule out cancer. After reading the report but not looking at the CT scan itself, the GI specialist indicated that this was a serious issue and needed to be resolved quickly. With that news, Robert became quite concerned. The gastroenterologist sent him to a surgeon for gallbladder removal. There was no cancer, and the gallbladder was perfectly normal. Robert still had the annoying pain in his back. At this point, he saw the gastroenterologist again, who listened more closely. He suggested Robert had acid reflux and prescribed a drug – Nexium, one of a category of drugs called a proton pump inhibitor, which prevents the stomach from making acid. Robert felt immediate relief. The answer was always there, but the PCP did not take the time to listen. The GI expert did not either until after the surgery. Moral: Think of horses when you hear hoof beats, not zebras. And most important, take a careful and thorough history.

But even when the diagnosis was determined, notice that Robert was given treatment for reflux in the form of a pill. The doctor did not mention simple lifestyle changes that might have been as effective – reduced caffeine and alcohol, waiting a few hours after dinner before going to bed, or raising the head of the bed four inches because it is harder for acid to run uphill. The doctor did not suggest Robert try to shed a few pounds. And there was defensive medicine here as well. The radiologist felt compelled to be cautious and then so did the gastroenterologist, and this led to a significant surgical procedure with discomfort, lost productivity, anxiety and costs to Robert and his insurer. Had the PCP spent more time in the first visit with Robert, it might have been clear that his symptoms were likely acid reflux, avoiding a long string of costly medical interventions.

Most of us go through life feeling fine, until one day something happens and then we call up the doctor. Is there a better way? A way that can keep us away from trips to the doctor for illness? A way that actually maintains wellness and health and avoids disease as much as possible? The short answer: yes.

We all want good health. But what does that require? It is more than seeing the doctor for an annual exam. It is a lifetime of specific behaviors, including diet, exercise, reduced stress, no smoking, good dental hygiene, wearing seat belts and not being distracted while driving. It is important to understand that we each need to take more direct responsibility for our own health and wellness. Attention to our behaviors is the key first step to lasting health and wellness. Having a good PCP is equally essential.

Everyone should have a primary care physician, particularly one well-schooled in current evidence-based care approaches yet attuned to the full gamut of integrative medical approaches such as chiropractic, nutrition, personal training, massage therapy and acupuncture. Your PCP should know you well and, through you, your family and how you fit into your community. You must be sure your primary care physician will spend the time needed to address health, wellness and disease. When there is an illness, you want a PCP who can be contacted readily, will spend the necessary time to make a correct and full diagnosis, and then create a beneficial management plan. Your PCP must offer you enough time to understand you and your needs. This is especially true if you have one or more chronic illnesses. But it is also important if you have a single, new acute problem that is slightly out of the ordinary – one that will take the doctor extra time to diagnose as he or she listens to your situation. Think back to the stories of Susan at the beginning of this book, Henry and his 20+ medications, and Robert at the start of this chapter. Each needed a PCP to listen thoroughly and when that did not happen, their care was far less than satisfactory. And unfortunately this happens all too often.

Since you, as a patient, are not the customer of the doctor in today's health-care system, you should take the initiative to change this paradigm. Paying the primary care physician directly means the physician will now become more attentive to your needs, allocate more time, listen carefully, work to under-stand a difficult issue and refer less to specialists. He or she can also offer more preventive care and take the time and energy to coordinate the care of chronic illnesses. In effect, you should ask to "buy" more time and attention than the PCP can offer based on your insurer's reimbursement rate. Direct payment changes the physician-patient relationship to a more normal and meaningful arrangement. If you have a high-deductible health policy and a health savings account (HSA), you will pay the doctor with tax-advantaged dollars.

You also must know that your PCP has an integrative type of practice. This does not mean that he or she uses or refers patients to complementary medicine approaches. Rather, it means the doctor is broad-minded and uses whatever well-proven techniques and approaches are beneficial to you. It means the PCP is not a "pill pusher," an aggressive test orderer or quick to send you to a specialist. Instead, it means the PCP spends the time needed to develop a diagnosis, recommend a lifestyle change and then add medical or surgical therapies as necessary. It means he or she is attuned to the medical home concept and accepts the role and responsibility for population health. This is the PCP who does not wait for you to visit the office but, working with a team, proactively reaches out to you for wellness, health maintenance and disease prevention.

Once you have the right PCP, is there anything you can do to receive the best possible health care? The PCPs that I interviewed suggested a few ideas that will make your doctor visits more effective. Keep a record in your wallet or purse of your medications and their dosages, your medical "ills" (what physicians call a "problem list"), and every provider you have seen recently and when. When you arrive at the office, be prepared with a list of issues you want to discuss. Put them in priority order. You do not want the most important issue to be fifth on your list, or it will be the one that you miss when the doctor must leave the exam room. And it is not a bad idea to have a copy of your list to hand to the doctor when you arrive so he or she can scan it and get an early idea of what the issues of the day will be.

Keep a copy of your medical record. Do not hesitate to ask your PCP for a copy – it is actually your property. Keep a copy of every laboratory test result, such as blood and urine tests, and a copy of every image taken, such as X-rays, CT scans, MRIs and ultrasounds, not just the reports. The CT scan or MRI can be easily downloaded to a CD or a memory stick by the radiology office at little or no charge. When you visit a specialist, he or she will (should) want to review the actual images, not just read the radiologist's report. It will save time and possibly even the need to repeat a test or X-ray. Ask for a copy of the specialist's written record. Take a copy to your PCP – the PCP may not have received it by the time you return for a visit.

If you are hospitalized, visit your PCP within 48 hours of discharge and bring a copy of the hospital discharge summary with you. Your PCP can then review your medications, post-hospital instructions and help you with any problems in the future. This is extremely important and could save you a return to the hospital.

Ask about using your PCP's personal cell phone number. Consider using email to request a prescription refill or ask a general question. But do not expect to use email for an acute or critical issue – call right away.

In my interviews, the PCPs suggested that the Internet can be both good and bad. There are large volumes of quality information available on the Internet, but there are just as many pages not founded on science. Use only high quality sources such as large academic medical center sites, the National Institutes of Health, and major charitable organizations such as the American Cancer Society or the American Heart Association.

You cannot change your genes, but you can affect the care of the body you were gifted at birth. Lifestyle changes are often important, and even at an advanced age, it is never too late to embrace preventive care. You need a good primary care physician, and your PCP must be someone who can give you the time you need. This usually means a doctor who has agreed to a smaller patient panel and fewer patient visits per day. In the short term, this may cost you a moderate fee, but it will be money well spent, especially if you and your doctor work together to maintain your wellness and health.

CHAPTER TWENTY

THE CHOICE IS YOURS:
A CALL TO ACTION

Dr. Digby has been a highly-regarded PCP by both patients and colleagues for more than 20 years. He had about 2,500 patients who he saw annually and another 1,000 who considered him their PCP even if they only came in for an unexpected acute episodic reason. He saw another 1,000 on occasion and was not certain if they considered him their PCP or if they found another doctor since the last visit. Dr. Digby was good at multitasking. He was efficient yet tried to never appear rushed despite seeing about 24 patients per day. He maintained his tradition of seeing his patients in the hospital when they were admitted and, whenever possible, he dropped by the ER if a patient was there. He also volunteered in a clinic one half-day per week. For many years, he shared night and weekend call with his partners, but more recently, he decided to handle his own patients and allowed them to call him seven days per week – he actually found this less stressful. But he felt run down. He was not dispirited by medicine, but he was frustrated by the requirements of insurers. They added no benefit to his patients and consumed his time, which could be better spent with the patients. He felt he earned a decent income, yet the price he paid in time and stress had become far too high to tolerate any longer.

He considered multiple approaches, including selling his practice to a local hospital, closing his practice entirely and accepting a non-clinical position at a nearby not-for-profit health care organization, or asking his patients to pay a yearly "administrative fee" that would offset uncompensated time after hours. He finally settled on converting his practice to a form of direct primary care. The process was somewhat painful, and many of his patients felt he was placing them at a disadvantage if they could not or chose not to pay the annual retainer. Others told him he was being unfair to them, and some suggested it was greed. Another group wished him well but would not pay the fee since they had insurance that already paid for primary care. As it turned out, about 500 patients signed up with his new practice arrangement. But he was surprised, he told me – some who he felt certain would stay with him did not, and others who he did not realize had a close tie to him chose to convert. He was particularly surprised (and annoyed) when a specialist physician who he had known for years asked for "professional courtesy" in lieu of the retainer payment.

Now a few years into his new practice, Dr. Digby is content, working hard, still seeing his patients in the hospital and ER, and providing what he feels is superior care to each patient. He is unencumbered by time constraints or the requirements of insurers. His patients are unified in their satisfaction. He and other PCPs like him have proven that "less means more" – or fewer patients means better care and quality.

Primary care needs to change. That change will need the concerted efforts of patients, doctors and other constituents. This may surprise you, but change will only happen when patients become outspoken advocates. It is worth the effort to get involved.

As you have heard me say throughout this book, primary care physicians need to care for fewer patients – not more – and should be able to earn an appropriate living at the same time. Fewer patients means more time for the patient and doctor to interact. It means more time for listening, building trust and healing. It means better diagnostics and improved treatment plans. It means fewer tests, X-rays, prescriptions and specialist visits. The result is better care, satisfied patients and doctors and dramatically reduced total costs of care. In order to drive down total healthcare costs while improving healthcare quality, we need to spend more money per patient for primary care.

Primary care, as it has been delivered for the past century, is rapidly transforming before our eyes. Many of the changes are quite disruptive. Some are for the good and some not so good. You and others like yourself can have a definitive impact on how primary care is practiced in the future. It can be practiced in a manner that offers superior care, a strong relationship between patient and doctor, and a reasonable price, all while dramatically reducing the total costs of care. This will require your active participation in the transition. The alternative – rushed visits, lack of a close doctor-patient relationship, an emphasis on specialty care and excessive prescription medications all lead to higher costs yet less quality.

Change will emanate only from the "front lines:" the doctors, nurse practitioners, physician assistants and others who provide primary care and their patients who demand a better deal. Solutions will not emanate from centralized planners mandating reforms. Innovation only occurs from those actually involved. In healthcare today, more decisions are made in a centralized way by well-meaning "experts" who have little or no idea about what it takes to provide real care to a real person by a real doctor. Once the centralized decision is made, it always requires many rules and regulations for implementation, which further impede progress, the doctor's autonomy, and the ability to innovate and improve the system.

This excerpt from an Op-Ed in the Baltimore Sun by long time geriatric focused primary care physician Andy Lazris, MD cuts to the heart of the issue. In it he is referring to the newly announced Medicare dictum that soon doctors "are paid not for visits and procedures but rather for the value of their work." Sounds good but "the truth is that we cannot measure quality. Medicare's quality indicators often diverge sharply from true quality geriatric care yet it is our compliance with those numbers that will now determine our salary. ...To Medicare and ACA reformers quality and value are broken down into discreet measurements that must be entered into a computer exactly as Medicare dictates....No wonder patients must face doctors who stare at computer screens and do not have time to listen....There is a better way forward....Eliminate the templates and scripted notes we have to complete, erase the erroneous measures of quality to which we are told to adhere, reduce the paperwork burdens needed to obtain health care and allow us to meaningfully care for our patients. ...Allow us in primary care to steer the ship. Enable us to treat patients as they want to be treated, to discuss with them the pros and cons of test and treatments, and to personalize care. Provide patients with choices: They can go to the hospital or get care at home for the same price; they can get an MRI for their back pain or have acupuncture treatment. It does not take a room full of experts and a book of rules, regulations and acronyms to fix our health care system. It takes common sense. Talk to practicing primary care doctors. You may learn something of real value."[62]

In primary care today, most of the innovation has come from individual primary care providers who decided to step away from the central planners, such as private insurance companies or the government, and work directly with patients. Free of the centralized bureaucratic regulations, they innovate with direct pay/retainer/membership/concierge models. They follow the precepts of the patient-centered medical home without worrying about the associated rules, regulations and documentation. Some are beginning to address population health in a proactive manner.

In this book, I advocate for direct primary care in one form or another because it is best for patients and primary care practitioners. Direct primary care allows the doctor the opportunity to give the type of outstanding care that each of us needs, including those who are currently healthy. Unfortunately, at present, direct primary care will not work for everyone. The three most common objections are the monthly or annual cost when one's current insurance (commercial or Medicare) already covers primary care, the often-incorrect assumption that the cost is too high and only for the wealthy, and patients are abandoned when a PCP converts his or her practice from 2,500 patients to less than one quarter that amount. We have discussed each of these issues and the advantages and disadvantages.

Although I advocate for direct patient care, many options can work. These approaches also create a reasonable PCP-to-patient ratio:

- Capitation, in which the PCP receives a large enough per-member per-month fee that the total number of patients drops from the current number. Recall the Erickson Living Medicare Advantage plan.
- Insurers change the fee-for-service reimbursement methodology to assure better care of chronic illnesses and enhanced preventive care, as we saw with CareFirst.
- Employers establish their own primary care operations with an appropriate employee-to-doctor ratio, as we saw with QuadMed, or pay for direct primary care via an HSA, as with Serigraph.

- Insurers decide to pay a monthly fee for direct primary care, as we saw with Nevada Health Co-op in association with Turntable Health, in which the usual requirements of insurers are waived in lieu of a fixed monthly payment.

- Insurers, employers, unions or associations contract with organizations like MedLion or Iora Health to provide primary care unencumbered by the usual insurance mandates, with only a reasonable number of patients per doctor depending on circumstances and with an emphasis on a team approach and health coaching.

- Insurers place extensive resources into primary care for the benefit of those with multiple chronic illnesses and socioeconomic deprivation, as is the case with the AbsoluteCARE contract with Amerigroup, a Medicaid managed care company.

TWO PATHS IN THE PRIMARY CARE ROAD TO THE FUTURE	
"Production Medicine" with High Patient-Doctor Ratio	*Comprehensive Extensive Primary Care With Low Patient-Doctor Ratio*
Frustrated Doctors and Patients	Satisfied Doctors and Patients Doctors with Time to Listen and Think
Over Utilization of Specialists Tests and Imaging Prescriptions ER Visits and Hospitalizations	Much Reduced Utilization of Specialists Tests and Imaging Prescriptions ER Visits and Hospitalizations
Primary Care Costs About 5 Percent of Total Costs	Primary Care Costs 50-100 Percent More
Continued High and Rising Total Costs of Care	Much Reduced Total Costs of Care With Slower Annual Rise

In each of these examples, the intention – whether stated or not – is to convert from a dysfunctional medical care delivery system to a true healthcare delivery system. When this happens, it is clear that the quality of care rises and the total costs decline, often dramatically. In each the key was innovation – stepping away from the current system and constructing a new, better approach.

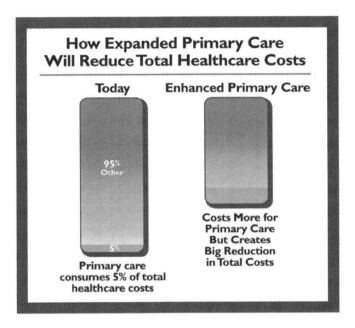

Innovation From the Bottom Up

Consider this analogy for the current health care conundrum: When an octopus settles on a coral reef, it changes colors to provide protection from predators. But the color changes are not directed centrally. Rather, each cell has the innate capacity to recognize its surroundings and change color to match. The octopus will end up with a well camouflaged body with each area colored appropriately for its immediate surroundings. We need that type of decentralized innovation in medicine today – innovation that starts with the provider and the patient.

Rather than centrally direct how healthcare delivery should be improved, we should assess the problem and determine the goal, which is to *create a primary care delivery system that offers high quality care to a satisfied patient by an enthusiastic and energized physician (or other provider) at a reasonable cost that lowers the total cost of care.* Then all who have the needed abilities and expertise can develop their own solutions to the problem. These individuals are at the front line, so they know better what will work in their setting. The solutions can be sorted out in the healthcare marketplace, with the best of each ultimately used together.

What has always driven individuals to become physicians, especially PCPs, is the opportunity for a trusting, meaningful and useful relationship with the patient. This relationship is the heart of primary care. The goal today should be to enhance that relationship by assuring that the PCP has the needed time with the patient for listening, thinking, preventing and coordinating. That means fewer patients per doctor and it means much less nonclinical busy work dictated by others. Another part of the goal is to reduce the burden on the PCP by making better use of the team. A third element is to assure a proactive approach with all patients at all times, not just when they show up at the office with a problem. When the PCP-patient relationship is present, the workload of the PCP is reduced, and the entire patient panel is proactively managed by the primary care provider and team, then the PCP becomes the backbone of the U.S. healthcare delivery system. This means assurance of excellent care, increased satisfaction for both provider and patient and reduced *total* costs of care. It means a *healthcare system,* not the medical care system as we have today.

The New Model for Primary Care

The new model for the delivery of primary care offers certain rights balanced by responsibilities for patient, provider and insurer alike.

BALANCING RIGHTS AND RESPONSIBILITIES		
	Rights	*Responsibilities*
Primary Care Doctor (PCP)	Fewer patients Less stress and frustration More time per patient Minimal time on non-clinical requirements Same income	Provide superior expanded comprehensive primary care that reduces total costs of care and includes: Team approach Proactive population health approach to care
Patient	Comprehensive primary care Relationship-based Patient-centric Trust with true healing	Pay extra (directly or indirectly) for comprehensive care
Insurer (Commercial or Governmental)	High quality care Reduced total costs of care	Pay PCP more per visit or per unit of time (PMPM) Or Pay the monthly/annual direct primary care membership fee/retainer
Employer	Healthy workforce Lower total costs of health care	Provide: Wellness programs Primary care with appropriate (low) employee-doctor ratio via Pay for in-house clinic Or Pay for direct primary care PCP retainer/membership Or Place money in HSA for direct primary care PCP

As a patient, you deserve a high level of care. The insurer and your employer want to see the total cost of health care come down. The physician wants the satisfaction of offering outstanding care, a reasonable income and a reasonable home life.

In return, the PCP has the responsibility of providing thorough care of patients. Thorough care includes being available on reasonable notice, with timing dependent on acuity. The patient visit should be long enough to fully assess and treat the problems, including underlying emotional anxiety and stress. The doctor must allocate sufficient time to listen and think. If there is a need for a specialist, the PCP should personally call and explain the reason for the referral and seek a prompt appointment. After the specialist visit, the PCP may need to reinforce and interpret the specialist's recommendations for the patient. When the patient's illness requires multiple specialists, the PCP needs to accept the role of coordinator of care (probably with assistance from an office team member) to ensure that each specialist is cognizant of the other's recommendations and that tests and prescriptions are neither duplicative nor will they lead to adverse interactions.

The PCP should also offer comprehensive preventive care, including advice about wellness and health, appropriate screening for treatable conditions and management of immunizations. In the process, it is appropriate to make the best use of community resources by encouraging use of the local senior center for intellectual stimulation, continuing education and socialization. Patients will likely need encouragement to eat a moderate Mediterranean diet, exercise regularly and stop smoking. The PCP must be cognizant of complementary medical techniques such as acupuncture for chronic pain, yoga and massage for stress, Reiki for energy balance, and chiropractic care for back and neck discomfort. The PCP should not do all of the counseling, training and coaching himself or herself – the practice team members and others should do most of this work.

Health promotion and disease prevention must not be left to the current approach of waiting for the patient to choose to visit the office. The doctor and his or her team should actively reach out to all of the patients in the practice. The team must determine who is at risk and then offer logical and intensive approaches for prevention and wellness maintenance. This might include a nutrition counselor, a personal trainer for exercise assistance and a smoking cessation counselor. A dedicated health coach can add high value to the equation. The team must take the same approach with those who already have a chronic illness. No longer can the healthcare team wait for the patient to call. Instead, they must create an in-house mechanism to stay in contact with the patients.

As a patient, you should be able to communicate as appropriate —by email, Skype or other digital means – and you should be able to call the PCP directly via cell phone during off hours if necessary.

Each encounter with the doctor's office should be positive. Customer service means a friendly face, a warm welcome, short waits for appointments and equally short waits in the "waiting room." Although sometimes the news from the doctor may not be positive, the experience should always be so.

With such a model, the PCP will practice in an integrative manner and, assuming he or she has the appropriate personality, will have a humanistic approach that engenders trust. Some physicians will reach the stage of true healers.

The insurer (and whoever pays the insurer such as employer, government or you) benefits with reduced *total* costs of care. You benefit with improved care and a meaningful relationship with your doctor. You will also benefit over time with reduced or stable health insurance premiums.

This sounds like a tall order but it is quite possible. They key is a payment model that is designed to ensure the PCP has the right number of patients and time to accomplish all of the above. At the same time, the payment model should force the physician to be accountable for the total health of each patient – population health. This means reorganizing the office team along the lines of the patient-centered medical home, although free of the burdens of unnecessary bureaucratic forms and checkboxes as is presently the case. It means assigning responsibility for data collection and entry, proactive population health approaches, preventive medicine, and chronic illness care coordination to the other clinicians on the team. By doing this, the PCP frees up time for complex issues and critical patient-PCP personal interaction, time to listen and time to think.

If this can be achieved with new models of reimbursement and a return to the old model of intense relationships with patients, then primary care will survive to drive the rest of the healthcare system to excellence at a much lower cost.

As a patient, the choice is yours. You have every right to quality care, but there is "no free lunch." The "right" to healthcare should not be interpreted to mean free healthcare. If you choose to select an insurance plan with a high deductible, you will save on premiums but will be responsible for paying for most of your primary care expenses out-of-pocket. You will be in a position to ask your doctor for more time since it is your money, and you will probably become more involved in your care by questioning recommendations and discussing plans with your PCP. Should you choose direct pay, a membership model or a retainer-based model for your primary care, it will cost more but it will offer more. If you choose a capitated program, you will gain more time with your PCP, but the insurer may narrow the network of specialists and hospitals available. The same goes for choosing a Medicare Advantage plan over Traditional Medicare. In the end, you must match your personal expenditures with your perception of your and your family's health care needs to choose what is best for your circumstances.

I am well aware that most Americans are not yet informed about the issues in primary care. Most do not realize how important and valuable true primary care can be to their health overall. Most people see primary care as for the "simple" problems and expect to see the PCP only episodically. A new paradigm is often difficult to embrace, but it is especially difficult when its purpose and logic are not appreciated. Americans have become used to an insurance model that purports to be prepaid medical care, and most of us are skeptical of stepping away from what we know. We are also not yet fully cognizant of the value of good preventive care. In addition, most are not familiar with the concept of population health or a proactive approach to managing health and wellness instead of only illness. All of these will need to sink into the collective consciousness before real change can occur.

The Solution or How to Achieve the New Primary Care Model

We must allow primary care physicians the *right* to care for fewer patients – 500-1,000 rather than 2,500-3,000 – yet retain an income equivalent to today. That means spending more money per patient for primary care. But to be cost neutral or cost advantageous, primary care physicians and effective teams must accept the *responsibility* to give that smaller number of patients outstanding health care, which will mean a much lower expense overall.

The government will not likely figure out a solution. Medicare, through its reimbursement policies over the years, has been the major cause of the crisis and typically deals with rising costs by instituting price controls. These have never worked and, in fact, have exacerbated the increasing costs of care.

The Affordable Care Act mandated a modest increase in primary care physician reimbursements by Medicare (10 percent) and by Medicaid (to Medicare levels), but this is too little, too late. Commercial insurers have generally followed Medicare's lead with reimbursements over the years, including the requirement to utilize the complex and yet inadequate coding systems called ICD-9 and soon ICD-10. Some examples, such as CareFirst/Blue Cross Blue Shield (Chapter 15) and the Erickson Living Medicare Advantage through United Healthcare (Chapter 15), have instituted creative and effective programs, but so far these are the exceptions. The advent of high deductibles, as encouraged by the ACA to bring down the premium levels, fits well with migrating to a direct primacy care physician's practice.

Returning to Lincoln's admonition, "Public sentiment is everything. With public sentiment, nothing can fail. Without it, nothing can succeed." When patients understand the value of comprehensive primary care, innovative change will surely follow.

I believe it will be mostly up to primary care physicians, in concert with their patients, to find their own solutions and change the paradigm of the care and business model. Physicians want to put patients first but circumstances have gotten in the way – bureaucracy, red tape, liability issues, and reduced reimbursements – all of which increase the costs of practice without improving care. The crisis in primary care needs to be solved if Americans are to have the level of care that they deserve – safe, equitable, accessible and high quality – and if the costs of that care are to ever become affordable.

A Call To Action
This is what each of the key participants in healthcare must do to solve the primary care crisis in the United States:

Insurance Executives
As an insurance executive (and by extension the employers, governments, unions, groups and individuals who pay the insurers' bills), your company

will benefit from developing models that encourage each PCP to have a more reasonable and justifiable patient panel size. This means paying the doctor more per patient encounter in the fee-for-service model, more per-member per-month in the capitation model or more in other organizational models of payment. Review the data available on how this approach will reduce hospitalizations and readmissions to the hospital while improving quality. Of course, if you grant more funds toward primary care, you will want an ironclad understanding that each patient will get the type of care needed and that, as a result, total costs of care will decline substantially.

Another approach, which may sound heretical to some but makes sense, is to pay the retainer or membership cost for the practice models that limit the patient panel and commit to team-based, population-type healthcare delivery. When conducted appropriately, they save you considerably. New entrants could do as well or better. Pair the retainer with a high-deductible catastrophic policy, as approved within the ACA. But do not expect or require mountains of paperwork to justify the retainer payment – that only pushes back toward the dysfunctional system at work today. Some requirements are appropriate: a limited number of patients, the team approach and population-type proactive practice management. Pay the retainer and step out of the way.

Why should the insurer pay for the retainer when insurance should be for the expensive and unexpected? This is not insurance; it is a fee for all primary care for a month or year. Paying the retainer aligns incentives to maintain wellness, detect chronic illnesses early and offer excellent yet inexpensive care. This saves you, the insurer, money – a lot of money. And your payers will be happy to save money on next year's premiums.

These retainer payments may increase the total dollars going toward primary care from the current 5-6 percent of all costs by one-half or perhaps double but with more than corresponding decreases in specialty and hospital care. The payments must vary so the PCP's panel size is appropriate for the population enrolled. Total numbers in the patient panel will vary depending on the individual demographics, with fewer patients if the population is mostly geriatric, for example.

Employers

You want your workforce to be healthy, productive and satisfied and you want to substantially reduce your expenses for employee health care. Today, most of your staff grumbles about the high cost of their share of the health care premium, yet many employees have or are at high risk for chronic illness, and your costs keep rising.

You need to make health a strategic company initiative as opposed to what today is probably a cost management or cost avoidance problem assigned to the HR department. The strategy needs to be elevated to the CEO and Board. You are in an excellent position to change the landscape and make primary care work for you and your company. You can force the change that is needed to assure that your employees get the time they need with the PCP so they receive outstanding primary care in a way that saves your company handsomely. I suggest you offer a high-deductible policy and an HSA, such as a consumer-directed health plan.

The CDHP is not enough by itself. Add to it. Offer your staff members who accept the CDHC a payment (for example, $1,000 for an individual and $2,000 for a family) toward the purchase of the annual (or monthly) retainer of a high-quality PCP who uses the direct primary care model. It will be a win-win for employer and employee.

Alternatively, contract with local PCPs to care for your employees and their families with a membership or retainer-based model, which you pay for directly. The doctor must agree to a limited number of patients, depending on the health demographics of your employees, with about 1,000 as an absolute maximum and fewer if you have staff with ongoing chronic illnesses. Insist that the PCPs practice in a team-based approach and address proactive population health, including extensive prevention, risk modification and chronic disease management.

As another approach, hire a company to develop a primary care program for you in a turnkey fashion. Require it to be organized so each PCP has an appropriate number of patients based on the health demographics of your workforce. Concurrently hire a firm to offer your employees sound wellness coaching and management and tie these two initiatives together to be seamless.

In any of these models, it is important that there is a real team approach, including health coaches, care coordination and proactive attention to each employee. Any of these will cost substantially more than typical episodic primary care and they will challenge you to spend more for primary care now, but the result will be a much healthier staff, greater productivity and insurance costs that stay flat or increase slowly. Your total costs will ultimately be much less, and both you and your employees will be more satisfied. It will be a good return on your investment.

Elected Officials

At first glance, you may be skeptical of comprehensive primary care because it costs more than typical care. But this is not the cost to focus on. The real measure is what the total cost of care? Expanded or comprehensive primary care as described in this book and exemplified by the many examples given does indeed cost more but the results is much reduced costs of care along with improved quality of care. This is what you want; it is worth advocating for it.

Improving primary care will mean a healthier society and superior quality at lower total costs overall. You should encourage insurance to combine a high deductible with catastrophic coverage. Policies should encourage insurers and self-insured employers to buy the retainer or to subtract the amount of the retainer from the deductible. Individuals should be able to own or transport their policies from job to job without fear of losing eligibility, and they should be able to pay for their coverage with tax-advantaged dollars, whether they buy it via their employer or via the individual market exchanges.

Those of limited means will need to have an assurance that they will not be bankrupted by a serious medical issue – the deductible needs to be lowered based on income. But the principle of one paying for their care directly either with their own money or with money placed in an HSA by government needs to be preserved. The individual needs to be directly responsible for payments.

Traditional Medicare should pay the membership or retainer for primary care practices that commit to a reasonable patient panel size, with Medicare-aged individuals on a panel of no more than about 500 members. This would save Medicare substantial money while ensuring superior care. But it is essential to recognize that paying the retainer is not the same as paying a reimbursement for a service with all of its attendant coding and billing necessities. It is a simple one-time payment with no other reporting requirements other than a certification from the PCP that he or she is giving full service primary care in a proactive, team-based manner with a limited number of patients under care.

Remember that innovation comes from the ground up, not the top down. Centralized planning and directives will continue to stifle meaningful improvements in health care delivery. Instead, set national goals, such as high-quality primary care, easy and full access, transparency in pricing, reduced total cost of care and higher overall quality and satisfaction. Then get out of the way. Avoid rules and regulations and encourage innovation by those on the front lines who can best understand the needs and the opportunities.

Various rules and regulations have been put in place for what may have seemed like logical reasons at the time but they have stifled the practice of medicine, especially primary care. Bureaucratic requirements that take away from patient care only lead to poorer care and greater expenses. Many PCPs are reacting by simply no longer participation in Medicare or Medicaid. It is time to take a close look at what regulation and requirements are really value added.

Government funding for specialty trainee slots at teaching hospitals should be reduced while funding for primary care is increased, meaning general pediatrics, general internal medicine and family medicine. There will be incredible pushback by the specialty societies and others but these combined steps will encourage more medical students to enter primary care rather than specialty care. Once students and trainees appreciate that they can give high quality care yet have a reasonable lifestyle and income, they will look to primary care as a career goal.

Academic Medical Center Leaders (Medical School Deans and Teaching Hospital CEOs)

You cannot be faulted for the basic non-sustainable business model that is actively destroying primary care. And you cannot directly fix it. But you can encourage students to enter primary care. You can also assure that students and residents have superb mentors and role models who are committed to the art of listening, developing trust with the patient, and teaching the fundamentals of solid preventive care and maintaining wellness rather than solely episodic medical care. Mentors who understand true healing and teach by example are rare and need to be cultivated. Mentors need to be honored and not denigrated because they spend much of their time outside of a research laboratory. You should ensure that mentors and role models teach the art of true healing and its importance to a solid therapeutic relationship.

You already want more students to enter primary care. Make sure they know about the options and the advantages of direct primary care. Invite practicing physicians in these models to address the class. Understanding that one can practice good quality medicine in a non-stressed atmosphere and with a decent income will encourage more students to consider primary care again as an acceptable career option.

You can also ensure that students, especially residents, are taught the elements of leading small groups, which will be found in the patient-centered medical home. In the process, students and residents need to appreciate the benefits of interdisciplinary care models and the value of working closely with nurse practitioners, physician assistants, nurses, pharmacists, social workers and others on a daily basis. This is best done as a regular part of the patient care environment, not in a lecture format. With this, teach the elements of integrative medicine and an appreciation for complementary medical modalities that have been proven to be efficacious. For many medical schools and teaching hospitals, this will be a major shift in emphasis, but it is a shift that must occur for primary care providers to practice medicine at the peak of their abilities and offer the type of proactive healthcare that their patients want and deserve.

You can also develop your own in-house primary care programs so the patient-to-doctor ratio is appropriate, unlike it is today. Your faculty should use the team model and engage in effective proactive population health. Of course, you are not reimbursed for this type of expansive primary care today, so you will need to advocate for new payment models. Seek support for limited patient panels and more time per visit from the local insurers. Not only will you manage their panels, but you will also teach the concepts and precepts to the next generation of physicians. Faculty who follow these principles with a limited panel of patients will be a strong example to students. It will show that primary care can be a professionally-rewarding career instead of one that is frustrating and lacking in satisfaction.

Corporations and entrepreneurs are demonstrating that they can deliver primary care in an effective, efficient manner. In general, academic medical centers do not do so but you could and you should. You should re-organize primary care practices with the team, interdisciplinary and proactive population health models. Traditionally, your faculty cares for some of the sickest of the sick. It would behoove you to look at what some companies are doing to advance care of these types of individuals by placing intense resources at the disposal of the PCP (such as care managers, health coaches, nutritionists, social workers, pharmacists, nurses and vans for patient transport) to manage only a reasonable number of patients' care in an interdisciplinary manner. Seek the help of insurers like Medicaid to fund your program at an enhanced PMPM rate with the proviso that you will reduce their total costs of care. It is good medicine and will teach the elements of team leadership and interdisciplinary care.

Finally, remember that it is a big step to go from residency to private practice. Students need education in the financial aspects of establishing a practice and an understanding of how the "system" works out in the real world away from the academic medical center or teaching hospital. And they need a general education in personal financial management, an education that they generally do not receive but need in order to function in the world at large.

Students and Trainees

If you have dreamed of being a primary care provider but become ambivalent as you learn about the frustrations and challenges of today's practice arrangements, then take some hope and re-evaluate. Join groups such as Primary Care Progress, which will teach you leadership and grassroots organizing skills. These are techniques you and your classmates can use to press your institution for curriculum changes and for honoring the professors who walk the talk. It will also help you to select an appropriate practice setting that fits your practice style and personal needs for family and home life.

Primary Care Physicians

You will be able to offer real healthcare rather than episodic medical care if you insist that you must care for a limited number of patients and give each patient the level of care you would want for yourself and your family members. Deep down, you want to put patient needs above all else. If you do using one of the approaches discussed in this book, you will have honored that commitment and you will find your own sense of satisfaction much improved and your frustration well reduced. Care can only the truly patient-centered if you have the time to offer comprehensive primary care. It is not about making your life better; it is about making the care of your patients better. But when that happens, you benefit markedly.

Up until now, most of you have just kept your head down and held your nose. But you really should take a leadership role; the issues are just too important to hope someone else will see the light and fix them. PCPs tend to avoid the political arena, but it would be useful for you to join and actively participate in your local medical society, the American Medical Association and your specialty college. There is strength in numbers. Politicians are good at counting the size and votes in a lobbying effort. Since the national organizations generally do not represent only primary care, other than the American Academy of Family Physicians, you may want to join forces with grassroots organizations that have emerged for this purpose, such as Primary Care Progress. You may also want to encourage your patients to be politically active through other organizations committed to enhanced health care rather than just episodic medical care.

Consider converting to a direct primary care practice in one of its various forms – direct pay or membership/retainer/concierge. Reduce your patient panel to 500-800 so you can offer same or next-day appointments, lengthy visits times, email and cell phone access. You will be more satisfied and your patients will be as well.

Alternatively, you could enter into agreements with insurers to offer care to fewer patients for a larger fee-per-visit or per-member per-month. If the insurer agrees, it will be undoubtedly with provisos that their total costs of care will come down as a result of your commitment to your patients' health.

You should also commit to avoiding unnecessary tests, images and pre-scriptions that are not clearly required on the basis of solid evidence. It is the physician's ethical responsibility to be appropriately parsimonious and not drive up medical costs.

Each patient should be afforded the time necessary for you to listen without unreasonable interruption and to reach well-founded decisions. You should also give each patient exemplary preventive care, with expanded attention and care coordination for those with chronic illnesses.

Reconsider how you organize your practice and your office. Assign more data entry tasks to others in the office and encourage all to work at their full capacity and training. Team-based care is relatively new, and teams require leaders to function at peak capacity. But physicians are usually not taught leadership in medical school or residency, so consider some training in team-based leadership. If you can develop adequate funding, consider following the general concepts of the medical home model and emulate the ideals of population health with proactive outreach to all patients in your panel on a regular basis. I recognize that this is an unprecedented change in how primary care has been delivered over the decades, and it requires a cultural and structural change in your practice that will be challenging but not overbearing.

If you accomplish this – and you can – you will once again become the healer that you originally sought to be when you entered medical school.

Individuals – Seeking Enhanced Healthcare Rather Than Episodic Medical Care

I saved you for last. You are the most important because change will only occur when individuals like yourself demand change. Inertia is still in full control. The critical tipping point has not yet been reached, but it could be with your added input.

You will benefit greatly from having a primary care physician, but it must be one who has the time and inclination to give you the care you deserve. Your PCP must have a limited number of patients and plenty of time for each patient visit. You may need to pay for this yourself.

Having a high-deductible insurance policy is a good first step. This means you will pay out-of-pocket for primary care but with just a portion of the money saved from your premiums. Now you will be the physician's direct customer. You should ask for whatever time you and the PCP need to resolve your issues effectively.

Better yet, look for a primary care physician who refuses insurance and accepts direct pay-per-visit with a reduced number of patients. You should ask to have the time you need for each visit. It will cost more, but it will be worth the price.

The best option, in my opinion, is to look (on these websites, for example**) for a doctor who accepts an annual retainer or membership for all care. It will cost you $750-$2,000 per year, but it will be money well spent. You will pay for it with your savings from purchasing a high-deductible insurance policy, and if you have an HSA, it will be with tax-advantaged dollars.

If you cannot obtain a high-deductible policy, including Medicare enrollees, you should decide if your healthcare priorities are high enough to justify the added costs of direct primary care to you and your family. It is fundamentally an issue of how you prioritize your health care needs relative to other needs. Balance the value of enhanced primary care with what you pay now for cable TV, your smartphone data plan, and trips to the movies.

For those of you who have no insurance, direct primary care may be the best way to obtain high-level care. You will pay out-of-pocket for the membership, but many DPC physicians find that individuals with no insurance make up a large proportion of their patients. The membership will cost you less than if you pay per visit to a local urgent care center or drug store clinic, and you will receive comprehensive relationship-based care, not just episodic care. In addition, the PCP will generally be able to eliminate or reduce your need to go to the expensive emergency room or urgent care center.

While selecting a direct primary care physician, learn if he or she has made arrangements for reduced-cost laboratory testing, reduced-cost radiology services and access to generic drugs at wholesale prices. DPC membership/retainer-based physicians take in new patients, so you should call and

---

** How do you find a direct primary care doctor? Ask your friends and colleagues who have a DPC doctor about their experiences with DPC and get references from them. Alternatively, go to services such as Direct Primary Care (www.dpcare.org) or American Academy of Private Physicians (www.privatephysicians.com), which can help link you with physicians who have a DPC practice in your area. Another excellent source is *Concierge Medicine Today*. You can also search online for direct primary care by including your state or a nearby city in the search.

check. You might be surprised to learn that vacancies exist. Patients leave the practice; some die, some move away. Find a doctor you like, and if the practice is full, get on the waiting list.

You may have a PCP who you really like even though he or she has too many patients and has to give too little time per visit. Tell your doctor about DPC (using this thorough summary, for example[††]) and encourage him or her to convert. Doctors are a "conservative" bunch – they are slow to embrace change unless it seems valuable and possible without stress and conflict. Only when patients understand DPC and clamor for its advantages will PCPs feel comfortable making the conversion.

Perhaps you and others in your company can convince your employer to pay for the retainer with the expectation that total costs of healthcare, including insurance, will be reduced.

It is also possible to receive this type of care through some – but certainly not most – capitated programs such as Medicare Advantage or commercial insurance. Check if the provider and the provider's insurer treat clients consistent with the principles I have described – fewer patients so the doctor can give each patient the time needed, same-day appointments, and immediate access to the physician 24/7 via cell phone. In addition, the PCP should pay careful attention to preventive care, care coordination and your emotional needs.

If you are over 65, look for a Medicare Advantage Program that gives the primary care physician a sufficiently high capitation rate (in dollars per-member per-month or year) and requires the doctors to have no more than 500 patients under care. Unfortunately, most of the insurers that offer Medicare Advantage programs still do not recognize the critical value of the primary care physician to both offer better quality care yet keep the total costs of care down. Most PCPs who accept Medicare Advantage patients today care for far too many patients to give the type of care I have advocated for here. You will need to shop with care.

[††] California Health Foundation has a thorough explanation and review of direct primary care, "On Retainer: Direct Primary Care Practices Bypass Insurance" written by Dave Chase and available at the Foundation website at http://bit.ly/1ELb36O or at www.directprimary-carejournal.com/store-books under White Papers.

Assuming you have selected a PCP using one of these approaches, you now will have a more direct professional relationship with your primary care physician. Still, you should insist on the following:

- prompt appointments,
- adequate visit time,
- a doctor who listens fully before making a diagnosis and recommending a treatment plan,
- a commitment to narrow the information gap between you and the PCP,
- thorough and intensive preventive care and wellness management,
- ready availability (same or next day) for episodic issues,
- enhanced comprehensive care of your chronic illnesses,
- coordination of your chronic illness care with other providers if needed,
- easy access with 24/7 cell phone,
- email and other digital venues for interaction,
- a well-functioning team approach that is proactive regarding preventive care, risk assessment and recognition/early management of chronic illnesses, and
- a personality and demonstrated ability that inspires your trust and the capacity to heal.

Combined, these reforms and steps will improve quality, increase satisfaction for all parties and reduce total health care expenditures. It will finally mean a *primary care system that offers high quality care to satisfied patients through enthusiastic and energized physicians at a reasonable price that lowers the total cost of care.*

The choice is yours. It is definitely true that you get what you pay for in healthcare. Unfortunately, today we often pay for not the best care at too high a price. Primary care does not need to be expensive, and comprehensive primary care should save considerable total dollars. But you should do the research before deciding. Think of it as an investment in your own health. What could be more important?

ACKNOWLEDGEMENTS

This book could never have come to fruition without the assistance and help of many individuals. Some of the most important are noted here.

Margaret Frazier converted my dictations to readable verbiage, fixed my grammar, proof read the entire manuscript, formatted it for publishing, checked each reference, and was critical to finding many of the patient stories.

Louis Moriconi (www.lmoriconi.com) used his superb professional graphic design skills to create the cover.

I am very grateful to economist Anirban Basu, Sage Strategy partners CEO for his on point Foreword that so well expresses the "crisis" in economic terms.

Many primary care physicians gave generously of their time for lengthy interviews about practicing primary care. Among them are: Kevin Carlson, MD, Delia Chiaramonte, MD, Richard Colgan, MD, Kisha Davis, MD, Louis Domenici, MD, Daniela Drake, MD, Alexa Faraday, MD, Michael Johnson, MD, John Hong, MD, Jon Izbicki, DO, Andy Lazris, MD, Gary Milles, MD, Carmen Nan, MD, Ryan Neuhofel, DO, Harry Oken, MD, Gary Prada, MD, Jerry Seals, MD, Marc Tanenbaum, MD, Josh Umbehr, DO, Andrew Wong, MD, and nurse practitioner Megan Schollenberger, NP.

Others interviews dealt with specific issues: Chet Burrell, CareFirst CEO, Garrison Bliss, MD, Qliance founder, Tom Blue, American Academy of Private Physicians chief strategy officer, Alan Cohn, Avesis chief executive,

Jeff Kane, MD, author, William Cossart, MedFirst Partners CEO, Dorothy Darby, Erickson Living Medicare Advantage plan administrator, Stephen Davis, MD, University of Maryland department of medicine chairman, James D'Orta, MD, Consumer Health Services, Inc. cofounder, Benjamin Edelman, MD, retired pathologist, Robert Enslein, McKay Shields LLC managing director, Walter Ettinger, MD, University of Maryland Medical System vice president for medical affairs, John Fairhall, Kaiser Health News senior editor, David Fogel, MD, Casey Health Institute co-founder, Gregory Foti, MD, AbsoluteCARE medical director, Kirk Gramoll, QuadMed vice president, Louis Grimmel, Lorien Health Systems chief executive, Jordan Grumet, MD, PCP and author *I Am Your Doctor*, Mark Hammett, Kelly Benefit Strategies, director of small group, Dan Hecht, MDVIP former CEO, Steven Horvitz, DO, The Institute For Medical Wellness, PCP in Moorestown, New Jersey, Margaret Kim, AllCareMD president, Andrea Klemes, DO, MDVIP medical director, Brian Klepper, WeCare principal and chief development officer, Thomas LaGrelius, MD, Skypark Preferred Family Care concierge physician, David Mayer, MD, MedStar Health SVP Quality and Safety, Andrew Morris-Singer, MD, Primary Care Progress president and co-founder, Matthew Narrett, MD, Erickson Living medical director, Michael Permenter, Private Practice Direct managing partner, Julien Pham, MD, MPH, RubiconMD founder and chief medical officer, James Pinckney II, MD, Diamond Physicians founder and CEO, Samir Qamar, MD, MedLion co-founder and CEO, Samuel Ross, MD, Bon Secours Baltimore Health System chief executive, Christopher Shoffner, Physician Care Direct chief risk officer, Andrew Schutzbank, MD MPH, Iora Health medical director and Primary Care Progress co-founder, Lucia Sommers, DrPH, University of California San Francisco professor, Michael Tetreault, *Concierge Medicine Today* editor, Brian Wheeler, CareFirst vice president.

Many individuals reviewed all or part of the manuscript as it was developing and offered important advice and encouragement. Among them are: Ronald Carlson, Health Care Financing Administration retired administrator, Dianne Connelly, PhD, Wisdom Well practitioner, Larry Gerrans, Sanovas, Inc. chief executive, Jon Izbicki, DO, primary care physician, Brian Kushnir, Added Value managing director, Michael Merson, former MedStar

Health president and Carefirst board chair, Matthew Taber, Medical Access Corporation of America chief operating officer, Josh Umbehr, DO, primary care physician and multiple consultants at Sage Growth Partners - Steven Brooks, MD, Chris DeMarco, Dan D'Orazio, Dana Kern, Don McDaniel, Robert McEwan and David McIntyre.

My literary agent, Cynthia Zigmund, Second City Publishing Services LLC, gave me excellent advice and direction as the book was in process, guided the proposal process and then the decision to use CreateSpace.

Carolyn Crist used her journalism skills to copy edit and smooth the text and reduce redundancies to make the manuscript read more smoothly.

Victor diPace, graphic designer at Sage Growth Partners, made the text more effective through his excellent infographic designs.

During the research for this book I placed questions on *LinkedIn* and posts at *KevinMD*. I am very appreciative of the many comments, pro and con, offered by readers.

Despite all this assistance, any errors are mine alone.

Most importantly, I offer my profound gratitude and thanks to my wife of 51+ years, Carol Schimpff, who has been always encouraging and committed to this project as it unfolded over the past three years.

ABOUT THE AUTHOR

Stephen C. Schimpff, MD FACP is an internist, researcher, professor of medicine and public policy, former University of Maryland Greenebaum Cancer Center director and former University of Maryland Medical Center chief executive officer. He is a graduate of Rutgers University and Yale School of Medicine. He is board certified in internal medicine, medical oncology and infectious diseases. Most of his career was spent at the National Cancer Institute, the University of Maryland Medical School and the University of Maryland Medical System. Since quasi-retirement he has authored four books for the general public on medical topics. He and Carol, his wife of over 50 years, live in Maryland.

Learn more about Dr. Schimpff's books, articles and blog at:
www.medicalmegatrends.com

ENDNOTES

1   Barnett, M, Song, Z, Landon, B. Trends in physician referrals in the United States, 1999-2009. *Arch Intern Med.* 2012;172(2):163-170. http://bit.ly/1ArJ2cr. Last accessed March, 2015

2   "Abraham Lincoln and public opinion," http://bit.ly/1Btpdqw. Last accessed March, 2015

3   Petterson, SM, Liaw, WR, Phillips, RL, Meyers, DS, Bazemore, AW. Projecting US primary care physician workforce needs: 2010-2025. *Ann Fam Med.* 2012;10(6):503-509. http://bit.ly/1C2rLvW Last accessed March, 2015

4   Lin, K. "We are spending billions to train the wrong kind of doctors," *KevinMD.com*, July 26, 2013, http://bit.ly/1DGeyrH. Last accessed March, 2015

5   Rosenthal, E. "Patient's costs skyrocket; specialists incomes soar," *New York Times*, January 18, 2014, http://nyti.ms/1GDaHN2. Last accessed March, 2015

6   Comparing the United States Healthcare to Other Developed Countries. http://bit.ly/1BFKtJi. Last accessed March, 2015

7   Woolf, SH and Landan, AY. The US health disadvantage relative to other high-income countries. *JAMA.* 2013;309(8):771-772. http://bit.ly/1ALRGCv Last accessed March, 2015

8   "A Survey of America's Physicians: Practice Patterns and Perspectives." *The Physicians Foundation*. http://bit.ly/1wJGJH0. Last accessed March, 2015

9   Kozel, M. "Understand the medical economics of a primary care practice," *KevinMD.com*, February 26, 2011, http://bit.ly/1AKtC7N. Last accessed March, 2015

10 Shanafelt, TD, Boone S, Tan L, et al. Burnout and satisfaction with work-life balance among US physicians relative to the general US population. *Arch Intern Med.* 2012;172(18):1377-1385. doi:10.1001/archinternmed.2012.3199. http://bit.ly/1BtuLBu. Last accessed March, 2015

11 Peckham, C. "Physician Lifestyles -- Linking to Burnout: A Medscape Survey," *Medscape.com*, March 28, 2013. http://bit.ly/1zPTrzn. Last accessed March, 2015

12 Beckman, H, Frankel, R. The effect of physician behavior on the collection of data. *Ann Intern Med.* 1984;101(5):692-696. http://bit.ly/1w7aMrm Last accessed March, 2015

13 Koven, S. "Is your doctor really present during your visit?," *KevinMD.com*, August 5, 2013, http://bit.ly/18cEArd. Last accessed March, 2015

14 Schimpff, S. The Future of Social Media in Healthcare, Foreword to Applying Social Media Technologies in Healthcare Environments, edited by C Thielst, HIMMS, Chicago, IL, 2014

15 Crow, R. "After residency, I'm scared to practice outpatient medicine," *KevinMD.com*, December 3, 2014. http://bit.ly/1zvkC6W. Last access March, 2015

16 The White Coat Ceremony was designed by The Arnold P. Gold Foundation in 1993 "to welcome entering medical students and help them to establish a psychological contract for the practice of medicine. The event emphasizes the importance of compassionate care for the patient as well as scientific proficiency.... At the ceremony, students are welcomed by their deans, the president of the hospital, or other respected leaders who represent the value system of the school and the new profession the students are about to enter. The cloaking with the white coats—the mantle of the medical profession—is a hands-on experience that underscores the bonding process. It is personally placed on each student's shoulders by individuals [often a physician relative] who believe in the students' ability to carry on the noble tradition of doctoring. It is a personally delivered gift of faith, confidence and compassion." Most medical schools now follow this tradition. More details at http://bit.ly/1A13W36. Last accessed March, 2015.

17 Curtis, J. "Beyond the white coat: training great doctors," *Yale Medicine*, Spring 2013. http://bit.ly/1aHeO0g. Last accessed March, 2015

18 Responses to a question posed by Paula Stanziani in the Healthcare Industry Professionals Group on LinkedIn "In one word what makes a great doctor?" November, 2013. The quoted section authored by Scott Sturtevant, ACHE.

19 Kane, Jeff. *The Bedside Manifesto Healing the Heart of Healthcare.* Cork: BookBaby, 2013.

20 Churchill, LR and Schenck, D. Healing skills for medical practice. *Ann Intern Med.* 2008;149(10):720-724. http://bit.ly/1Dq9OE7 and a beautiful blog post by Dr. Sharon Orrange, "What makes a physician a healer?," *Daily Strength.org*, November 21, 2008. http://bit.ly/1BMMWSz Both last accessed March, 2015

21 Guarneri, Mimi. *The Heart Speaks: A Cardiologist Reveals the Secret Language of Healing.* New York: Simon & Schuster, 2006.

22 Upledger, J. "Self-discovery and Self-healing." In *Healers on Healing*, edited by R. Carlson, Los Angeles: J.P. Tarcher, 1989.

23 Colgan, Richard. *Advice to the Healer on the Art of Caring.* 2nd ed. New York: Springer, 2013.

24 Wikipedia, http://bit.ly/1FKzm17. Last accessed March, 2015

25 25 Remen, Rachel Naomi. *My Grandfather's Blessings: Stories of Strength, Refuge, and Belonging.* New York: Riverhead Books, 2000.

26 Sir Luke Fildes (1843-1927), The Doctor, Exhibited 1891, Oil on Canvas, ©Tate, London, 2015 Used with permission

27 Lazris, A. *Curing Medicare: One Doctor's View of How Our Health Care System Is Failing the Elderly and How to Fix It.* CreateSpace, 2014.

28 Baron, RJ. What's keeping us so busy in primary care? A snapshot from one practice. *N Engl J Med.* 2010;362:1632-1636. http://bit.ly/1M0MyRz. Last accessed March, 2015

29 Altschuler, J, Margolius, D, Bodenheimer, T and Grumback, K. Estimating a reasonable patient panel size for primary care physicians with team-based delegation. *Ann Fam Med.* 2012;10(5)396-400. http://bit.ly/1AXPtYe. Last accessed March, 2015

30 Sommers, LS, and J. Launer, eds. *Clinical Uncertainty in Primary Care the Challenge of Collaborative Engagement.* New York, NY: Springer, 2013.

31 Donelan, K, DesRoches, C, Dittus, R, Buerhaus, P. Perspectives of physicians and nurse practitioners on primary care practice. *N Engl J Med.*

2013;368:1898-1906. http://bit.ly/1AeSMa4 Last accessed March, 2015

32   Sedillo, R. "Nurse practitioners belong in the primary care movement," *primarycareprogress.com, Progress Notes*, October 23, 2014. http://bit.ly/1zPX0FT. Last accessed March, 2015

33   The National Committee for Quality Assurance (NCQA) has developed guidelines for the Patient Centered Medical Home and the process by which physicians can apply for certification http://bit.ly/1wEdS10. Last accessed March, 2015

34   Betbeze, P. "How the medical home may save primary care," *healthleadersmedia.com*, September, 2013. http://bit.ly/1wABvNt. Last accessed March, 2015

35   Backer, LA. The medical home: an idea whose time has come ...again. *Fam Pract Manag.* 2007;14(8):38-41. http://bit.ly/1AXWmsL. Last accessed March, 2015

36   Friedberg, MW, Schneider, EC, Rosenthal, MD, Volpe, KG and Werner, RM. Association between participation in a multipayer medical home intervention and changes in quality, utilization and costs of care. *JAMA.* 2014;311(8):815-825. http://bit.ly/1EYiB2g. *Last accessed March 2015*

37   Schwenk, TL. The patient centered medical home: one size does not fit all. *JAMA.* 2014;311(8):802-803. http://bit.ly/1Fe95s8 *Last accessed March 2015*

38   Kernisan, L. "Primary care doctors need 35 hour work weeks," *KevinMD.com*, July 11, 2013, http://bit.ly/1aHqZKi. Last accessed November 1, 2013

39   Hodach, R. ACOs and population health management: How physician practices must change to effectively manage patient populations. American Medical Group Association. http://bit.ly/1CCdTtQ. *Last accessed March 2015*

40   "2014 Survey of America's physicians, practice patterns and perspectives." *The Physicians Foundation.* http://bit.ly/1M11Ojm. Last accessed January 26, 2014

41   Peckham, C. "Medscape internist lifestyle report 2015," *medscape.com*. http://bit.ly/1ERkcJv. Last accessed March, 2015 but available only to Medscape members

42 *The Big Bang Theory* clip of "thinking," https://www.youtube.com/watch?v=i5oc-70Fby4. Last accessed March, 2015

43 Wiebe, C. "What would you change about medicine, Medscape survey, Experts weigh in," *medscape.com*. October 24, 2013, http://bit.ly/17WqoCT. Last accessed March, 2015 but available only to Medscape members

44 Wickline, S. "10 Questions: Steven Horvitz, DO," *medpagetoday.com*, March 20, 2014, http://bit.ly/1N5KqeK. Last accessed March, 2015

45 Young, RA, Bayles, B, Hill, J, Kaparaboyna, K and Burge, S, Family physicians' opinions on the primary care documentation, coding and billing system, Family Medicine, 2014; 46: 378-384 http://bit.ly/18cSr0M. Last accessed March, 2015

46 Malaspina, P. "A presidential apology to the medical profession," Presidential address to the Erie County, NY Medical Society, *generalsurgerynews.com*, November 13, 2013.

47 Schiff, G., et al. Primary care closed claims experience of Massachusetts malpractice insurers. *JAMA Intern Med.* 2013;173(22):2063-2068. http://bit.ly/18lQfUN Last accessed March, 2015

48 Grumet, J. "Are physicians becoming distracted drivers," *inmyhumbleopinion.blogspot.com*, April 27, 2014, http://bit.ly/1BOvrD5. Last accessed March, 2015

49 "The most common gripes patients have about their doctors," *huffingtonpost.com*, January 17, 2014 http://huff.to/1wEsPAi. Last accessed March, 2015

50 The Associated Press-NORC Center for Public Affairs Research, "Finding Quality Doctors: How Americans Evaluate Provider Quality in the United States," May-June, 2014 http://bit.ly/1GDoiE3. Last accessed March, 2015

51 Wible, P. "The #1 thing patients want from doctors," *idealmedicalcare.org/blog*, February 1, 2015, http://bit.ly/1BOvJd6. Last accessed March, 2015

52 McGinnis, J and Foege, W. Actual causes of death in the United States. *JAMA.* 1993;270(18):2207-2212. http://bit.ly/1zQkMl9. Last accessed March, 2015

53 Jones, D, Podolsky, M, and Greene, J. The burden of disease and the changing task of medicine. *N Engl J Med.* 2012;366:2333-2338. http://bit.ly/1G7u2sl. Last accessed March, 2015

54   Mokdad, AH, Marks, JS, Stroup, DF, and Gerberding, JL. Actual causes of death in the United States, 2000. *JAMA.* 2004;291(10):1238-1245. http://bit.ly/1M0Ne9H. Last accessed March, 2015

55   DeVol, R and Bedroussian, A, with Charuworn, A, Chatterjee, A, Kim, IK, Kim, S and Klowden, K. Milken Report on Chronic Illnesses. "An Unhealthy America: The Economic Burden of Chronic Disease," 2007. http://www.milkeninstitute.org/publications/view/321 Last accessed March, 2015

56   Dentzer, S. One payer's attempt to spur primary care doctors to form new medical homes. *Health Affairs.* 2012;31:341-349. http://bit. ly/1AYiIKB. Last accessed March, 2015

57   Health, United States, 2013, Centers for Disease Control, National Center for Health Statistics, 2014   http://www.cdc.gov/nchs/ Last accessed March, 2015

58   Brody, H. Medicine's ethical responsibility for health care reform — the top five list. *N Engl J Med.* 2010;362:283-285. http://bit.ly/1AYj18d. Last accessed March, 2015

59   "Medical Anamnestics," *A Country Doctor Writes:,* April 4 and May 2, 2014, http://acountrydoctorwrites.wordpress.com/   Last accessed March, 2015

60   ICD-10 is a diagnostic coding system established some years ago by the World Health Organization (WHO) and is just being introduced into the United States. The older system called ICD-9 had 13,600 codes; the newer ICD-10 has 69,000. All hospitals and doctors and most other providers will have to use these codes in order to be reimbursed by commercial or governmental insurers. The older coding system, for example, might have identified a condition of the ovary whereas the new system will differentiate right, left, both or unspecified. In the case of a fracture, the new code will differentiate, for example, an initial visit for a fracture, a follow-up for a healing normally fracture, follow-up with nonunion or mal-union, or follow-up for late effects of a fracture. Etc. Although systematic and straight forward, it is a safe bet that learning the new system will take some substantial time. It will be one more thing that a small office of one or a few PCPs can expect will limit productivity. A cottage industry has developed to teach and help

implement the new system. No other country uses ICD-10 as the basis for billing and reimbursement.

61   Cutler, D, and Ghosh, K. The potential for costs savings through bundled episode payments. *N Engl J Med.* 2012;366:1075-1077. http://bit.ly/1ALUT55. Last accessed March, 2015

62   Burwell, S. Setting value-based payment goals – HHS efforts to improve U.S. Health Care. *N Engl J Med.* 2015;372:897-899. http://bit.ly/1N5Wr3J. Last accessed March, 2015

63   Lazris, A. "Medicare 'quality indicators' diverge from quality care," *Baltimore Sun, Op-Ed*, January 29, 2015, http://bsun.md/1BOEaoI. Last accessed March, 2015

64   I Love Lucy chocolate conveyor belt segment. http://bit.ly/1DqT5k0 Last accessed March, 2015

65   *Concierge Medicine Today.* http://bit.ly/1AYl2kM. Last accessed March, 2015

66   Chesanow, N. "Cash only practice: what you need to do to succeed," *Medscape Business of Medicine*, July 24, 2013. http://bit.ly/1DQvJnY. Last accessed March, 2015 but available only to Medscape members

67   Schimpff, S. "Health Care Fix: Patients Pay Doctors." *Washington Times, Op-Ed.* October 16, 2012. http://bit.ly/1G7yyXH. Last accessed March, 2015.

68   Kaiser Family Foundation 2013 employer health benefits survey, August, 2014. http://bit.ly/1N5XD7l. Last accessed March, 2015

69   Personal communication, Representative of Patient Care Direct, North Carolina

70   Henderson, M. As part of a comment to a post on *KevinMD.com* by Dr. Josh Umbehr. Available at http://bit.ly/1wF30zV. Last accessed March, 2015

71   Willis, K, personal communication and Atlantic Integrated Health, http://www.aihinc.com Last accessed March, 2015

72   Neuhauser, A. "Physicians abandon insurance for 'blue collar' concierge model," *US News and World Report*, April 1, 2014 . http://bit.ly/18BDaHO. Last accessed March, 2015

73   Izbicki, J, Personal communication, April 21, 2014

74 Epstein, J. "The Obamacare revolt: physicians fight back against bureaucratization of health care," *reason.com*, March, 2013, http://bit.ly/1N5YqoS. Last accessed March, 2015

75 Neuhofel, R, Personal communication, April 22, 2014

76 A word of caution to the doctor who is reading this book and contemplating the switch; get expert advice and guidance in advance. There are companies that specialize in this area. Find a firm that can assist with the transition to make it not only compliant with local, state and national regulations but smooth and less painful for both doctor and patient; not a bad idea considering all of the issues and sensibilities that can be involved. Organizing the appropriate letters, town hall meetings, reorganization of the PCP's office, etc. can be an unnerving proposition, all the more so for a busy doctor. Organizations like Concierge Medicine Today and the American Academy of Private Physicians can offer guidance. Alternatively, seek out a physician who has already made the conversion and get detailed advice. Having assistance is essential.

77 Klemes, A, Seligmann, R, Allen, L, Kubica, M, Warth, K and Kaminetsky, B. Personalized preventive care leads to significant reductions in hospital utilization. *Am J Manag Care*. 2012;18(12):e453-e460. http://bit.ly/1GDKwFY. Last accessed March, 2015

78 Seligmann, RE, Gassner, LP, Stolzberg ND, Samarasekera, NK, Warth, K, and Klemes, A. A personalized preventive care model versus a traditional practice: comparison of HEDIS measures. *International Journal of Person Centered Medicine*, 2012;2:775-779. http://bit.ly/1ALb9bd. Last accessed March, 2015

79 Bliss, G, Personal Communication from the founder of Qliance, September 7, 2014

80 Bliss, E. "Qliance: New primary care model delivers 20 percent lower overall healthcare costs, increases patient satisfaction and delivers better care," *PR Newswire*, January 15, 2015. http://prn.to/17IAHKH. Last accessed March, 2015

81 Knutson, R, Gryta, T, and Kendall, B. "Brewing Telecom Deals Bring Long-Promised Future Into View" *Wall Street Journal*, May 5, 2014. The WSJ requires a subscription to access this article. http://on.wsj.com/1DQghs7. Last access March, 2015

82 Martinez, W and Gallagher, TH. Ethical concierge Medicine? In *Virtual Mentor*; *AMA Journal of Ethics*. 2013;15(7):576-580. http://bit.ly/1Dr00tr. Last accessed March, 2015

83 Bessemer, J. Quoted in *Concierge Medicine Today*, May 1, 2014. http://bit.ly/1AYl2kM. Last accessed March, 2015

84 Burrell, C. Personal communication, 2011

85 Dentzer, S. "One payer's attempt to spur primary care doctors to form new medical homes," *health affairs*.org, 2012; 31: 341-349. http://bit.ly/1AYiIKB. Last accessed March, 2015

86 Tocknell, M. "CareFirst boasts $136m in savings on PCMH," *HealthLeadersMedia*, June 12, 2013

87 Wheeler, B. Personal communication, April, 2014

88 Morris-Singer, A. Interview, June 4, 2014

89 Lazris, A. Personal Communication, February 4, 2015 and the PCAC website http://www.primarycareaction.com/. Last accessed March, 2015

90 Foti, G. Personal Communication as part of a tour of AbsoluteCARE in Baltimore, April 2, 2014

91 Gwande, A. "The hot spotters: can we lower medical costs by giving the neediest patients better care?," *The New Yorker*, January 24, 2011

92 Jonas, M. Healing health care - Do Bob Master and Rushika Fernandopulle have the cure for what ails American medicine? *Commonwealth Magazine*, Winter 2014. http://bit.ly/1K4vo9W. Last accessed March, 2015

93 Schutzbank, A. Personal communication, May 9, 2014

94 "The CEOs' top priorities," *Wall Street Journal*, November 24, 2013. http://on.wsj.com/1AMlSgX Last accessed March, 2015 Requires subscription

95 Merrill, R and Merrill, JG, An evaluation of a comprehensive, incentivized worksite health promotion program with a health coaching component, International Journal of Workplace Health Management, 2014, 7: pp.74 – 88 Abstract available at http://bit.ly/1wWAjUY. Last accessed March, 2015 Required payment

96 Gramoll, K, and Heberer, J. Personal communication, July 8, 2014

97   Enterprise risk management, 3 part monograph, American Society for Healthcare Risk Management of the American Hospital Association, 2006 Available at www.ashrm.org under resources

98   Torinus, John. *The Grassroots Health Care Revolution How Companies across America Are Dramatically Cutting Their Health Care Costs While Improving Care*. New York: BenBella Books, 2014.

99   Umbehr, J. "A solution to ER overcrowding: direct care," *KevinMD.com*, April 30, 2014, http://bit.ly/1GDNUAD. Last accessed March, 2015

INDEX